Keto So Cookbook

Keto soups and stews easy recipes. 101+ Low carb recipes, rapid to cook, ready to eat in few minutes, perfect for fat burning!

Author : **Caren Larsen**

Table Of Content

Introduction

These days it seems like everyone is talking about the ketogenic (in short, keto) diet - the very low-carbohydrate, moderate protein, a high-fat eating plan that transforms your body into a fat-burning machine. Hollywood stars and professional athletes have publicly touted this diet's benefits, from losing weight, lowering blood sugar, fighting inflammation, reducing cancer risk, increasing energy, to slowing down aging. So, is keto something that you should consider taking on? The following will explain what this diet is all about, the pros and cons, as well as the problems to look out for.

Chapter One

What Is Keto?

Normally, the body uses glucose as the main source of fuel for energy. When you are on a keto diet and you are eating very few carbs with only moderate amounts of protein (excess protein can be converted to carbs), your body switches its fuel supply to run mostly on fat. The liver produces ketones (a type of fatty acid) from fat. These ketones become a fuel source for the body, especially the brain which consumes plenty of energy and can run on either glucose or ketones.

When, the body produces ketones, it enters a metabolic state called ketosis. Fasting is the easiest way to achieve ketosis. When you are fasting or eating very few carbs and only moderate amounts of protein, your body turns to burn stored fat for fuel. That is why people tend to lose more weight on the keto diet.

Benefits of The Keto Diet

The keto diet is not new. It started being used in the 1920s as a medical therapy to treat epilepsy in children, but when anti-epileptic drugs came to the market, the diet fell into obscurity until recently. Given its success in reducing the number of seizures in epileptic patients, more and more research is being done on the ability of the diet to treat a range of neurologic disorders and other types of chronic illnesses.

Neurodegenerative diseases. New research indicates the benefits of keto in Alzheimer's, Parkinson's, autism, and multiple sclerosis (MS). It may also be protective of traumatic brain injury and stroke. One theory for keto's neuroprotective effects is that the ketones produced during ketosis provide additional fuel to brain cells, which may help those cells resist the damage from inflammation caused by these diseases.

Obesity and weight loss. If you are trying to lose weight, the keto diet is very effective as it helps to access and shed your body fat. Constant hunger is the biggest issue when you try to lose weight. The keto diet helps avoid this problem because reducing carb consumption and increasing fat intake promote satiety, making it easier for people to adhere to the diet. In a study, obese test subjects lost double the amount of weight within 24 weeks going on a low-carb diet (20.7 lbs) compared to the group on a low-fat diet (10.5 lbs.).

Type 2 diabetes. Apart from weight loss, the keto diet also helps enhance insulin sensitivity, which is ideal for anyone with type 2 diabetes. In a study published in Nutrition & Metabolism, researchers noted that diabetics who ate low-carb keto diets were able to significantly reduce their dependence on diabetes medication and may even reverse it eventually. Additionally, it improves other health markers such as lowering triglyceride and LDL (bad) cholesterol and raising HDL (good) cholesterol.

Cancer. Most people are not aware that cancer cells' main fuel is glucose. That means eating the right diet may help suppress cancer growth. Since the keto diet is very low in carbs, it deprives the cancer cells of their primary source of fuel, which is sugar. When the body produces ketones, the healthy cells can use that as energy but not the cancer cells, so they are effectively being starved to death. As early as 1987, studies on keto diets have already demonstrated reduced tumor growth and improved survival for several cancers.

Comparing Standard American, Paleo, & Keto Diets

(As a % of total caloric intake)

	Carbs	Protein	Fat
Standard American Diet	40-60%	15-30%	15-40%
Paleo Diet	20-40%	20-35%	25-50%
Keto Diet	5-10%	10-15%	70-80%

The key distinction between the keto diet and the standard American or Paleo diets is that it contains far fewer carbs and much more fat. The keto diet results in ketosis with circulating ketones ranging from 0.5-5.0 mm This can be measured using home blood ketone monitor with ketone test strips. (Please know that testing ketones in the urine are not accurate.)

How to Formulate A Keto Diet?

1. Carbohydrates

For most people, to achieve ketosis (getting ketones above 0.5 mM) requires them to restrict carbs somewhere between 20-50 grams (g)/day. The actual amount of carbs will vary from person to person. Generally, the more insulin resistant a person is, the more resistant they are to ketosis. Some insulin-sensitive athletes exercising vigorously can consume more than 50 g/day and remain in ketosis, whereas individuals with type 2 diabetes and insulin resistance may need to be closer to 20-30 g/day.

When calculating carbs, one is allowed to use net carbs, meaning total carbs minus fiber and sugar alcohols. The concept of net carbs is to incorporate only carbs that increase blood sugar and insulin. Fiber does not have any metabolic or hormonal impact and so do most sugar alcohols. The exception is maltitol, which can have a non-trivial impact on blood sugar and insulin. Therefore, if maltitol is on the ingredient list, sugar alcohol should not be deducted from total carbs.

The level of carbs one can consumes and remain in ketosis may also change over time depending on keto-adaptation, weight loss, exercise habits, medications, etc. Therefore, one should measure his/her ketone levels on a routine basis.

In terms of the overall diet, carb-dense foods like pasta, cereals, potatoes, rice, beans, sugary sweets, sodas, juices, and beer are not suitable.

Most dairy products contain carbs in the form of lactose (milk sugar). However, some have fewer carbs and can be used regularly. These include hard cheeses (Parmesan, cheddar), soft, high-fat cheeses (Brie), full-fat cream cheese, heavy whipping cream, and sour cream.

A carb level less than 50 g/day generally breaks down to the following:

5-10 g carbs from protein-based foods. Eggs, cheese, and shellfish will carry a few residual grams of carbs from natural sources and added marinades and spices.

10-15 g carbs from non-starchy vegetables.

5-10 g carbs from nuts/seeds. Most nuts contain 5-6 g carbs per ounce.

5-10 g carbs from fruits such as berries, olives, tomatoes, and avocados.

5-10 g carbs from miscellaneous sources such as low-carb desserts, high-fat dressings, or drinks with very small amounts of sugar.

Beverages

Most people require at least half a gallon of total fluid per day. The best sources are filtered water, organic coffee and tea (regular and decaf, unsweetened), and unsweetened almond and coconut milk.

Diet sodas and drinks are best avoided as they contain artificial sweeteners. If you drink red or white wine, limit to 1-2 glasses, the dryer the better. If you drink spirits, avoid the sweetened mixed drinks.

2. Protein

A keto diet is, not a high protein diet. The reason is that protein increases insulin and can be converted to glucose through a process called gluconeogenesis, hence, inhibiting ketosis. However, a keto diet should not be too low in protein either as it can lead to loss of muscle tissue and function.

The average adult requires about 0.8-1.5 g per kilogram (kg) of lean body mass per day. It is important to make the calculation based on lean body mass, not total body weight. The reason is that fat mass does not require protein to maintain, only the lean muscle mass.

For example, if an individual weigh 150 lbs. (or 150/2.2 = 68.18 kg) and has a body fat content of 20% (or lean body mass of 80% = 68.18 kg x 0.8 = 54.55 kg), the protein requirement may range from 44 (= 54.55 x 0.8) to 82 (= 54.55 x 1.5) g/day.

Those who are insulin resistant or doing the keto diet for therapeutic reasons (cancer, epilepsy, etc.) should aim to be closer to the lower protein limit. The higher limit is for those who are very active or athletic. For everyone else who is using the keto diet for weight loss or other health benefits, the amount of daily protein can be somewhere in between.

Best sources of high-quality protein include:

- Organic, pastured eggs (6-8 g of protein/egg)
- Grass-fed meats (6-9 g of protein/oz)
- Animal-based sources of omega-3 fats, such as wild-caught Alaskan salmon, sardines, and anchovies, and herrings. (6-9 g of protein/oz)
- Nuts and seeds, such as macadamia, almonds, pecans, flax, hemp, and sesame seeds. (4-8 g of protein/quarter cup)
- Vegetables (1-2 g of protein/oz)

3. Fat

Having figured out the exact amounts of carbs and protein to eat, the rest of the diet comes from fat. A keto diet is necessarily high in fat. If sufficient fat is eaten, body weight is maintained. If weight loss is desired, one should consume less dietary fat and rely on stored body fat for energy expenditure instead.

(As a % of total caloric intake)

_____Maintain   Weight_____Lose Weight

Carbs_____5-10%_____5-10%

Protein_____10-15%_____10-15%

Fat from diet_____70-80%_____35-40%

Fat from stored body fat___0%_____35-40%

For individuals who consume 2,000 calories a day to maintain their weight, daily fat intakes range from about 156-178 g/day. For large or very active individuals with high energy requirements who are maintaining weight, fat intakes may even exceed 300 g/day.

Most people can tolerate high intakes of fat, but certain conditions such as gallbladder removal may affect the amount of fat that can be consumed at a single meal. In which case, more frequent meals or use of bile salts or pancreatic enzymes high in lipase may be helpful.

Avoid eating undesirable fats such as trans-fat, highly refined polyunsaturated vegetable oils, as well as high amounts of omega-6 polyunsaturated fats.

Best foods to obtain high-quality fats include:

- Avocados and avocado oil

- Coconuts and coconut oil

- Grass-fed butter, ghee, and beef fat

- Organic, pastured heavy cream

- Olive oil

- Lard from pastured pigs

- Medium-chain triglycerides (MCTs)

MCT is a specific type of fat that is metabolized differently from regular long-chain fatty acids. The liver can use MCTs to rapidly-produce energy, even before glucose, thus allowing increased production of ketones.

Concentrated sources of MCT oil are available as supplements. Many people use them to help achieve ketosis. The only food that is uniquely high in MCTs is coconut oil. About two-thirds of the coconut fat is derived from MCT.

Who Should Be Cautious with A Keto Diet?

For most people, a keto diet is very safe. However, certain individuals need to take special care and discuss with their doctors before going on such a diet.

Those taking medications for diabetes. Dosage may need to be adjusted as blood sugar goes down with a low-carb diet.

Those taking medications for high blood pressure. Dosage may need to be adjusted as blood pressure goes down with a low-carb diet.

Those who are breastfeeding should not go on a very strict low-carb diet as the body can lose about 30 g of carbs per day via the milk. Therefore, have at least 50 g of carbs per day while breastfeeding.

Those with kidney disease should consult with their doctors before doing a keto diet.

Common Concerns with A Keto Diet

Not being able to reach ketosis. Make sure you are not eating too much protein and there are no hidden carbs in the packaged foods that you consume.

Eating the wrong kinds of fat such as the highly refined polyunsaturated corn and soybean oils.

Symptoms of a "keto-flu," such as feeling light-headed, dizziness, headaches, fatigue, brain fog, and constipation. When in ketosis, the body tends to excrete more sodium. If one is not getting enough sodium from the diet, symptoms of a keto-flu may appear. This is easily remedied by drinking 2 cups of broth (with added salt) per day. If you exercise vigorously or the sweat rate is high, you may need to add back even more sodium.

Dawn effect. Normal fasting blood sugars are less than 100 mg/dl and most people in ketosis will achieve this level if they are not diabetic. However, in some people fasting blood sugars tend to increase, especially in the morning, while on a keto diet. This is called the "dawn effect" and is due to the normal circadian rise in morning cortisol (stress hormone) that stimulates the liver to make more glucose. If this happens, make sure you are not consuming excessive protein at dinner and not too close to bedtime. Stress and poor sleep can also lead to higher cortisol levels. If you are insulin resistant, you may also need more time to achieve ketosis.

Low athletic performance. Keto-adaptation usually takes for about 4 weeks. During which, instead of doing intense workouts or training, switch to something less vigorous. After the adaptation period, athletic performance usually returns to normal or even better, especially for endurance sports.

Keto-rash is not a common side effect of the diet. Probable causes include the production of acetone (a form of ketone) in the sweat that irritates the skin or nutrient deficiencies including protein or minerals. Shower immediately after exercise and make sure you eat nutrient-dense whole foods.

Ketoacidosis. This is a very rare condition that occurs when blood ketone levels go above 15 mM. A well-formulated keto diet does not cause ketoacidosis. Certain conditions such as type 1 diabetes, being on medications with SGLT-2 inhibitors for type 2 diabetes, or breastfeeding require extra caution. Symptoms include lethargy, nausea, vomiting, and rapid shallow breathing. Mild cases can be resolved using sodium bicarbonate mixed with diluted orange or apple juice. Severe symptoms require prompt medical attention.

Is Keto Safe for Long-Term?

This is a area of controversy. Though there have not been any studies indicating any adverse long-term effects of being on a keto diet, many experts now believe that the body may develop a "resistance" to the benefits of ketosis unless one regularly cycles in and out of it. Also, eating a very high-fat diet in the long-term may not be suitable for all body types.

Cyclical keto diet

Once you can generate over 0.5 mM of ketones in the blood consistently, it is time to start reintroducing carbs back into the diet. Instead of eating merely 20-50 g of carbs/day, you may want to increase it to 100-150 g on those carb-feeding days. Typically, 2-3 times a week will be sufficient. Ideally, this is also done on strength training days on which you increase your protein intake.

This approach of cycling may make the diet plan more acceptable to some people who are reluctant to permanently eliminate some of their favorite foods. However, it may also lower resolve and commitment to the keto diet or trigger binges in susceptible individuals.

HOW TO MAKE KETO CHICKEN SOUP WITH CAULIFLOWER RICE

- I was excited to try this Keto Chicken Soup. I've used cauliflower rice as a side and addition to salads, but I've never tried it in the soup. It was awesome. It added just the right amount of flavor and texture, so you truly don't miss the rice.

- Here's how to make the cauliflower rice: Cut the cauliflower in half and remove as much of the stem and leaves as possible. Then, cut the cauliflower into small florets removing any of the remaining stems. Place the cauliflower florets in a food processor or blender and pulse just until the cauliflower is broken down into small rice-sized pieces.

- If you don't have a food processor or blender, grate the cauliflower on the large holes of a box grater after cutting in half and removing the stems and leaves.

- You can also use purchased fresh or frozen cauliflower rice to save time!

- From there, this Keto Chicken Soup with cauliflower rice is super simple to make: Just sauté the onion and celery and then add in the aromatics. This will help bring out the flavor of the garlic, thyme, and paprika.

- Then stir in the broth and then add the chicken and rice cauliflower and simmer until cooked through.

- To turn this keto chicken and cauliflower rice into a low-carb chicken noodle soup, just replace the cauliflower rice with low-carb noodles of your choice! I love the idea of adding zucchini noodles!

- It's ready in just over 30 minutes. I love the gorgeous orangish-red color and subtle flavor the paprika adds and the chunks of chicken thighs are tender and perfect. It is surprisingly flavorful.

- We added on some parsley for a bit of color, but feel free to omit it if you don't have any on hand.

WHY SOUPS & STEWS ARE THE PERFECT KETO FOOD

- They're simple, easy and adaptable. If you're new to the Keto diet or cooking in general soups are a great place to start. Don't have this or want to add a little more of that... go for it.

- They're economical. The Keto diet can be expensive with its emphasis on organic protein, but soups and stews allow you to stretch your ingredients.

- They're quick. There are not many pre-made convenience foods available on the Keto diet, but many soups and stews can be ready in under 40 minutes making them the perfect weeknight dinner.

- They're great for meal-prep and make ahead meals. Make them ahead and then pack them up for the perfect lunch on the go.

- They're scalable. Have, a big family... double the recipe. Cooking for just yourself... then make half. Most of these recipes can be adjusted very easily.

- They're accessible. No weird ingredients you've never heard of or will never be able to find. You'll be familiar with all of the ingredients, which will be comforting when you are adjusting your nutritional plan.

- They're healthy. This is the most important one. All of these recipes are chocked full of beneficial nutrients. Especially if you make your broth!

This cookbook is great even if you aren't following a Keto or low carb diet. Seriously, who doesn't want a book filled with healthy and flavorful soups that your whole family will love!

Going Keto: Why It's Good for You

Keto diets have come on strong in the past year and a half and for good reason. It's a great way to not only shed those unwanted pounds quick but also a great way to get healthy and stay that way. For those that have tried the Keto Diet and are still on it; it's more than just a diet. It's a way of life, a completely new lifestyle. But like any major shift in our lives, it is not an easy one, it takes an incredible amount of commitment and determination.

Good for Some But not for all? - Although a ketogenic diet has been used to greatly improve people's quality of life, there are some out there who do not share the majority's way of thinking. But why is that exactly? Ever since we can remember we have been taught that the only way to get rid of the extra weight was to quit eating the fat-filled foods that we are so accustomed to eating every day. So instructing people to eat healthy fats (The keyword is Healthy) you can certainly understand why some people would be skeptical as to how and why you would eat more fat to achieve weight loss and achieve it fast. This concept goes against everything we have ever known about weight loss.

How Keto Started - Discovered by endocrinologist Rollin Woodyatt in 1921 when he found that 3 water-soluble compounds Accenture, B-hydroxybutyrate and Acetoacetate (Known together as Ketone bodies) were produced by the liver as a result of starvation or if the person followed a diet rich with high fat and very low carbs. Later on that year a man from the Mayo Clinic by the name of Russel Wilder named it the "Ketogenic Diet," and used it to treat epilepsy in young children with great success. But because of advancements in medicine, it was replaced.

My Struggles Starting Keto - I started Keto February 28th, 2018, I had attempted the Keto Diet once before about 6 months prior but was never able to make it through the first week. The first week on Keto is the worst part of the entire process; this is when the dreaded Keto Flu appears also called the carb flu. The Keto Flu is a natural reaction your body undergoes when switching from burning glucose (sugar) as energy to burning fat instead. Many people who have gone on the Keto Diet say that it feels similar to withdrawing from an addictive substance. This can last anywhere between 3 days to an entire week, it only lasted a few days in my case.

People who have had the keto Flu report feeling drowsy, achy, nauseous, dizzy and have terrible migraines among other things. The first week is usually when people attempting a Keto Diet fail and quit, just remember that this happens to everyone early in the process and if you can get past the first week the hardest part is over. There are a few remedies you can use to help you get through this rough spell. Taking Electrolyte supplements, staying hydrated, drinking bone broth, eating more meat and getting plenty of sleep. Keto Flu is an unfortunate event that occurs to everyone as the body expels the typical day-to-day diet. You just have to power through.

What Does A Ketogenic Diet Look Like? - When the average person eats a meal rich in carbs, their body takes those carbs and converts them into glucose for fuel. Glucose is the body's main source of fuel when carbs are present in the body, on a Keto diet there are very low if any at all carbs consumed which forces the body to utilize other forms of energy to keep the body functioning properly. This is where healthy fats come into play, with the absence of carbs the liver takes fatty acids in the body and converts them into ketone bodies.

An ideal Keto diet should consist of:

• 70-80% Fat

• 20-25% Protein

• 5-10% Carbs

You should not be eating more than 20g of carbs per day to maintain the typical Ketogenic diet. I ate less than 10g per day for a more drastic experience but I achieved my initial goals and then some. I lost 28 lbs. in a little under 3 weeks.

What Is Ketosis? - When the body is fueled completely by fat it enters a state called "Ketosis," which is a natural state for the body. After all of the sugars and unhealthy fats have been removed from the body during the first couple of weeks, the body is now free to run on healthy fats. Ketosis has many potential benefits-related to rapid weight loss, health or performance. In certain situations, like type 1 diabetes excessive ketosis can become extremely dangerous, whereas in certain cases paired with intermittent fasting can be extremely beneficial for people suffering from type 2 diabetes. Substantial work is being conducted on this topic by Dr. Jason Fung M.D. (Nephrologist) of the Intensive Dietary Management Program.

What I Can and Can't Eat - For someone new to Keto it can be very challenging to stick to a low-carb diet, even though fat is the cornerstone of this diet you should not be eating any kinds of fat. Healthy fats are essential, but what is healthy fat you might ask. Healthy fats would consist of of grass-fed meats, (lamb, beef, goat, venison), wild-caught fish and seafood, pastured pork & poultries. Eggs and salt-free butter can also be ingested. Be sure to stay away from starchy vegetables, fruit, and grains. Processed foods are in no way accepted in any shape or form on the Ketogenic diet, artificial sweeteners and milk can also pose a serious issue.

Why the Keto Diet Is So Effective for People Over 50?

The keto diet has gained popularity in recent years and has become a nutritional plan favored by individuals of all ages. That said, this dietary roadmap might precipitate particularly important health benefits to persons over age 50.

Keto Diet Overview

Scientifically classified the ketogenic diet, this nutritional plan stresses the decreased consumption of foods containing carbohydrates and a increased intake of fats. The reduced intake of carbohydrates is said to eventually place the bodies of participating dieters into a biological and metabolic process known as ketosis.

Once ketosis is established, medical researchers opine the body becomes especially efficient in burning fat and turning said substances into energy. Moreover, during this process, the body is thought to metabolize fat into chemicals categorized as ketones, which are also said to provide significant energy sources.

[An accelerator of this is an intermittent fasting method where the restricting of carbs causes your body to access the next available energy source or ketones that are derived from stored fat. In this absence of glucose, fat is now burned by the body for energy.]

There are several other specific ketogenic diets including:

Targeted (TKD)

 Those is participating in this version gradually add small amounts of carbohydrates into their diet.

Cyclical (CKD)

 Adherents to this dietary plan consume carbohydrates on a cyclical basis like every few days or weeks.

High-Protein

High-protein diet observers consume greater quantities of protein as part of their dietary plans.

Standard (SKD)

Typically, this most commonly practiced version of the diet intake significantly diminished concentrations of carbohydrates (perhaps as little as five percent of all dietary consumption), along with protein-laden foods and a high quantity of fat products (in some cases, as much as 75 percent of all dietary needs).

In most cases, the average dieter or someone new to the keto diet partakes in the standard or high-protein versions. The cyclical and targeted variations are usually undertaken by professional athletes or persons with very specific dietary requirements.

Recommended Foods

Keto diet adherents are encouraged to consume foods like meat, fatty fishes, dairy products such as cheeses, milk, butter and cream, eggs, produce products possessing low carbohydrate concentrations, condiments like salt, pepper and a host of other spices, various needs, and seeds and oils like olive and coconut. On the other hand, certain foods should be avoided or strictly limited. Said items include beans and legumes, many fruits, edibles with high sugar contents, alcohol, and grain products.

Keto Diet Benefits to Individuals Over 50

Keto diet adherents, especially those aged 50 and older, are said to enjoy numerous potential health benefits including:

Increased Physical and Mental Energy

As people grow older, energy levels might drop for a variety of biological and environmental reasons. Keto diet adherents often witness a boost in strength and vitality. One reason said occurrence happens is because the body is burning excess fat, which in turn gets synthesized into energy. Furthermore, systemic synthesis of ketones tends to increase brain power and stimulate cognitive functions like focus and memory.

Improved Sleep

Individuals tend to sleep less as they age. Keto dieters often gain more from exercise programs and become tired easier. Said occurrence could precipitate longer and more fruitful periods of rest.

Metabolism

Aging individuals often experience a slower metabolism than they did during their younger days. Long-time keto dieters experience a greater regulation of blood sugar, which can increase their metabolic rates.

Weight Loss

Faster and more efficient metabolism of fat helps the body eliminate accumulated body fat, which could precipitate the shedding of excess pounds. Additionally, adherents are also believed to experience a reduced appetite, which could lead to diminished caloric intake.

Keeping the weight off is important especially as adults age when they may need fewer calories daily compared to when living in their 20s or 30s even. Yet it is still important to get nutrient-rich food from this diet for older adults.

Since is common for aging adults to lose muscle and strength, a high protein-specific ketogenic diet may be recommended by a nutritionist.

Protection Against Specific Illnesses

Keto dieters over age 50 could reduce their risk of developing ailments such as diabetes, mental disorders like Alzheimer's, various cardiovascular maladies, various kinds of cancer, Parkinson's Disease, Non-Alcoholic Fatty Liver Disease (NAFLD) and multiple sclerosis.

Aging

Aging is considered by some as the most important risk factor for human illnesses or disease. So, reducing aging is the logical step to minimize these risk factors of disease.

Good news extending from the technical description of the ketosis process presented earlier, shows the increased energy of youth as a result and because of the usage of fat as a fuel source, the body can go through a process where it can misinterpret signs so that the mTOR signal is suppressed and a lack of glucose is evident whereby it is reported aging may be slowed.

Generally, for years, multiple studies have noted that caloric restriction can aid in slowing aging and even increase lifespan. With the ketogenic diet, it is possible, without reducing calories to affect anti-aging. An intermittent fasting method used with the keto diet can also affect vascular aging.

When a person fasts intermittently or when on the keto diet, BHB or Beta-Hydroxybutyrate is produced that is believed to induce anti-aging effects.

To be fair, as reported in the US National Library of Medicine National Institutes of Health article "Effects of Ketogenic Diets on Cardiovascular Risk Factors" in May 2017; the ketogenic diets, which are very low in carbohydrates and usually high in fats and/or proteins are used effectively in weight loss during treatment of obesity and cardiovascular diseases. However, an important note in the article was that "Results regarding the impact of such diets on cardiovascular risk factors are controversial" and "Moreover, these

diets are not safe and can be associated with some adverse events.
"

Safe to say, more is needed than simply researching this diet, benefits, positive effects, and side effects especially in aging adults by the internet and periodicals alone. One specifically should consult her or his medical professional about specific concerns.

Chapter Two
99+ keto soups and stews

Leftover Steak Soup

You can make this easy low carb soup recipe in no time at all! Use leftover steak if you have it, or cook up some fresh sirloin. You will not regret it!

Leftover steak recipes that taste Brand NEW!

Beef Stew & a few other leftover steak recipes they'll beg for!

Don't throw away your leftover beef; you can use it in another mouth-watering meal. If you have a large family the ability to use leftovers is really important. It's even better if you know what to do with them so they truly are a "new" meal instead of a warmed-over version of the day before!

- 1 lb steak
- 1/4 c sweet onion
- 1/4 c olive oil
- 32 oz V8 juice low sodium
- 16 oz water
- 1 c peas
- 1 c potato

- 1 c carrots
- 2 bay leaves
- 1/4 c freshly chopped parsley
- 2 tsp kitchen bouquet
- 2 c noodles

- Saute onion in olive oil in a skillet.
- Add V8 juice, water and all other ingredients except noodles.
- Simmer 1 1/2 hours until slightly reduced.
- Add noodles simmer additional 30 minutes.
- Serve with warm cornbread and fresh coleslaw.

A terrific brunch recipe:

- sliced or cubed pieces of leftover steak
- 1 green pepper diced
- 1 red pepper diced
- 1/8 c sweet onion finely chopped
- 6 organic eggs beaten
- 3/4 c heavy cream
- dash of cumin
- 1 c cubed pieces of day-old or tough bread

Grease pan places bread pieces on the bottom. Combine all other ingredients stirring slightly to combine. Pour over bread and bake for 20 minutes or till slightly golden and cooked through. Serve immediately with sliced organic tomatoes and sourdough or potato bread toast.

Curried Pumpkin Soup

This Pumpkin Curry Soup from Carolyn Ketchum's cookbook "Keto Soups & Stews" is so perfect for warming you up on a cool Fall day. I made the dairy-free version which was so rich and creamy using coconut milk. Can you believe this is ready in 20 minutes and has only 5.4 net carbs?!

You can opt to come up with your pumpkin soup recipes or better still borrow from friends or browse on the internet. Pumpkin soup is simply made by combining the broth or stock with the meat of a blended pumpkin. This is not the only item on pumpkin soup recipes but it is correct to say that they are the main ingredients.

There are various kinds of pumpkin soups and they all come with there sets of ingredients and the recipe to be followed. In this case, we are going to talk about the curried pumpkin soup recipe. As for the ingredients you will need to peel two cloves of garlic, one med onion, 1 gram jalapeno pepper, and coarsely chopped, two stalks of celery cut into two-inch length, carrots, 2 tbsp. Olive oil, 3 c low salt chicken stock, one bay leaf, curry powder, turmeric, a pinch of cayenne pepper, salt to add taste, fresh ground pepper, 1/4 c shelled raw pumpkin seeds, 2 tbsp. flat-leaf parsley chopped, 1 tbsp. Sour cream [optional] and of course pumpkins, after all, it's a pumpkin soup recipe.

Know that the ingredients for the pumpkin soup recipes are all in place, you should first place the garlic a food processor, pulse until chopped, put the onions and pulse until they are chopped then set aside. Put celery in the food processor until chopped then add jalapeno for the same process then put them aside. Do the same for the carrots and then set aside. Know that the recipe is already underway; you should proceed by heating 1 tbsp. of the Olive oil at a medium heat followed by adding onion and garlic. You should stir occasionally for about six minutes. Add carrots, celery, and jalapeno and fry lightly in a pan for 5 minutes. Then add the pumpkins and the rest of the pumpkin soup recipes. Have them boil then reduce the heat until the vegetables are tenderly cooked for about 8 minutes.

On the saute pan, you should be heating one tbsp. on the remaining Olive oil one, a medium heat then adds the pumpkin seeds and the remaining 1/2 tsp. of salt and cook for around 30 seconds. Remember you should be shaking the pan constantly to avoid burning. The process should go on until all the pumpkin seeds have popped. After the results are achieved, you should remove the seeds then you add parsley.

For the wind-up, you ought to place the two cups of the vegetable that has been cooked and the 1/2 cup liquid that is in the bowl of the processor then puree until the results are smooth. Then you place the puree back into the pumpkin soup and stir. Stir in the sour cream and remember to adjust the seasoning if it will be desired. Afterward, add the roasted pumpkin seeds stir gently and your pumpkin soup recipe will be ready to serve.

Instant Pot chicken soup

This Instant Pot chicken soup is so simple and hearty with lots of veggies. Make it creamy, but still healthy and low carb with the addition of a little heavy cream. Chicken Soup Brings Back Memories

Looking back on our childhoods many of us will remember our mothers making chicken soup for us when we were sick. Those are some great memories. Any time that we would get sick mom was off to the kitchen to start a pot of chicken soup. Memories of childhood are precious for most of us and the smell of chicken soup wafting through the house warms us to our very core. I had pneumonia recently and yearned for a bowl of mom's chicken soup, so when I recovered and my daughter got sick I was at the stove preparing a pot of chicken noodle soup. If you would like to share your fondest memory place it under the comment section and share it with others.

For most of you reading this, you grew up eating chicken noodle soup and while I love chicken noodle soup I thought I would share with you my chicken and rice soup recipe and one of my chicken noodle soup recipes. Just a precursor to the recipes, you can substitute noodles for rice and vice versa. Here is a little piece of advice, when using a recipe follow the directions the first time and when you make it again, change it up, add one of your favorite spices or if it is a fish recipe with a sauce try your favorite fish the next time, don't worry if it doesn't turn out, we all have failures and successes. I play around with recipes all the time and because I know how to blend spices and flavors, I have more success.

Chicken Soup Recipes

- Italian Chicken and Rice Soup

- 2-3 tablespoons Olive Oil

- 6 ounces Pancetta (or regular bacon) chopped

- 1 large onion (medium dice)

- 2-3 large carrots

- 2-3 stalks celery

- 4 cloves garlic

- 3 bay leaves

- 1/2 tsp saffron threads

- 2 lbs boneless skinless chicken breast

- 16 ounces chicken stock (made from 2 tablespoons chicken base and 2 cups water) This is better than chicken stock from a can or a box.

- 1 cup long-grain rice (I use wild rice that I have let soak overnight)

- 1/2 ground pepper

Directions:

Heat oil in a medium to the large stockpot. Add pancetta (or bacon) and cook until lightly browned. Add onion, carrots, celery and cook until onion is translucent. Add garlic, bay leaves, and saffron; cook for 45 seconds.

Add chicken and chicken broth, turn heat up to medium-high, cover and cook 15 minutes or until chicken is no longer pink. remove chicken and allow it to cool enough that you can touch it, shred chicken. Add rice and pepper, cook for 25-30 minutes. Return chicken to the pot and cook until chicken is hot.

 Remove bay leaves and serve.

Chicken Noodle Soup

- 3 tablespoons olive oil

- 1 large onion

- 5 stalks celery sliced

- 5 carrots sliced

- 4 garlic cloves minced

- 3 bay leaves

- 1 1/2 teaspoons poultry seasoning

- 1 1/2 teaspoons coriander seeds crushed

- 1/2 teaspoon nutmeg

- 4 cups chicken broth (made from 8 tablespoons chicken base and 4 cups water)

- 1 1/2 pounds chicken breast

- 1 package Reames noodles or 1 package egg noodles

Directions:

Heat oil in a large stockpot. Add onions and garlic cook until onion is translucent. Add carrots and celery cook 8 minutes. Add all seasonings cook 30 seconds. Add chicken and broth increase heat to medium-high. Bring almost to a boil, partially cover and cook for 15 minutes or until chicken is no longer pink. Remove chicken and allow it to cool. Shred chicken and return to pot. Add noodles cook for 8-10 minutes. Remove and discard the bay leaves.

Ready to serve.

When you are sick and feeling miserable you want comfort food and chicken soup always brings comfort. I hope that you try these chicken soup recipes and they bring you comfort on a cold, dreary day or a day when nothing will make you feel better until you have some of mom's homemade chicken soup.

Cream of Cauliflower Soup with Curry

Just like the fashion industry, the food industry has its trends. What's trending now? These vegetables are grabbing the limelight--Brussels sprouts, kale, and cauliflower. Recipes for these vegetables are popping up everywhere, on the Internet, in magazines, newspapers, and even conversation. If you haven't tried this trio before, you may be hesitant to do so.

But your grandmother and mother were right when they proclaimed, "Eat your vegetables. They're good for you!" Vegetables contain vitamins and minerals that are essential for good health.

According to the Self Nutrition Data website, cauliflower contains 25 calories per serving, three grams of fiber, two grams of sugar, and two grams of protein. It also contains vitamins A, C, K, folate, calcium, magnesium, phosphorus, and potassium.

My husband loves raw cauliflower and likes crisp slices of it in salat. Recently I bought a head-on sale and discovered the reason for the reduced price. The vegetable was starting to get soft. Since I coulddon't put it in a salad, I thought about mashing it like potatoes. Then I thought of soup. I live in Minnesota and its winter, with wind chills that can go as low as 41 below zero. Soup sounded mighty good.

Cauliflower and curry go well together, so I added some to the soup. If you don't like this spice leave it out. If you love this spice add more. Cooking the curry for a minute before adding the other ingredients brings out its flavor. After the vegetables are done, the mixture is purred with a hand blender. You may also use a stand blender, but I use a hand one because it's safer. I don't have to pour hot soup into a glass container and can puree the soup right in the pot.

I garnished the soup with garlic and butter croutons, but other flavors would taste good too. Here is my recipe for Cream of Cauliflower Soup with Curry.

INGREDIENTS

- 1 tablespoon olive oil

- 1 tablespoon butter

- 1 tablespoon curry powder

- 1 medium yellow onion, chopped

- 1 rib celery, chopped

- 1 cup baby carrots, cut into 1/2-inch chunks

- 1 carton (32 ounces) salt-free chicken broth

- 1 cup of water

- 1 chicken bouillon cube

- 3/4 medium head cauliflower, cut into small pieces

- 8 ounces Neufchatel cheese, room temperature

- 3 tablespoons Italian parsley, chopped (for garnish)

- Packaged croutons (for garnish)

METHOD

Put olive oil and butter in a soup pot. As soon as the butter has melted, stir in curry powder and cook 1 minute. Add onion, celery, and carrots and cook until vegetables are soft, about 10 minutes. Add cauliflower, cover, and bring to a boil. Reduce heat and simmer for 15 minutes. Turn off heat and stir in Neufchatel cheese. Remove pot from heat. Puree mixture with a hand blender. Garnish with chopped parsley and croutons, or omit them and serve the soup with crusty bread. This recipe freezes well.

Albondigas Soup

Albondigas Soup is a hearty Mexican meatball soup with a simple soup base made of diced tomatoes, chipotle salsa, and broth.

Albondigas Soup is a delicacy that originated in Spain and is loved equally in the realm of Latin America. However, that doesn't mean that you won't like it if you are not from any of those countries. Maybe you already have, and you just don't know it yet. Albondigas, when translated to English, would mean "meatball." This dish is perfect for a meatball lover and can be quite filling. The preparation time isn't all that long and the dish itself doesn't require a whole lot more effort than your average soup. However, the result is a whole lot better and tastier than any average soup.

There are variations to this dish as there are in most dishes but the variations involve more of an addition of ingredients than replacements. All the same, you might want to think about how to make this dish special for your taste buds as you could easily do so if you wanted.

Preparation Time of Albondigas

- Preparation Time: 20 Minutes

- Serving time: 40 Minutes

- Ingredients for preparing Albondigas

- Diced and Peeled Potatoes (Small) - 2

- Sliced Carrots - 4

- Water - 1 Quart

- Diced Onion - 1

- Beef Bouillon Cubes - 2

- Salsa (Medium or Hot) - 1 1/2 Cups

- Ground Beef - 1 1/2 Pounds

- Milk - 1/3 Cup

- Seasoned Dry Bread Crumbs - 1/3 cup

- Chopped Cilantro (optional)

Directions to prepare Albondigas

1. Get a large stockpot ready and add water, potatoes, carrots, salsa, onion, and the bouillon cubes as well. Bring, the mix to a boil, and reduce to a medium simmer. Stir the mix occasionally for around ten minutes.

2. Mix the breadcrumbs, milk, and beef in a separate bowl. Form into meatballs of your desired size and drop carefully into the broth which should be boiling by now. Once it does boil again, reduce the heat further.

3. Cover the pot and allow cooking for 15-20 minutes. Once you are satisfied with the tenderness of vegetables is to your liking, remove from heat and serve after sprinkling some chopped cilantro if you wish. Enjoy your Albondigas!

Nutrition Value of Albondigas

Major Nutrition Content for Albondigas:

• Cholesterol

• Sodium

• Carbohydrates

• Dietary Fiber

• Protein

Total Calorie Value per Serving: 326 Calories

Total Servings: 6

It isn't very odd if you have already started having ideas about how to make the soup taste better or maybe personalize it a bit more to your liking. Either way, do feel free to share your thoughts with us and help us make some better or more varied Albondigas.

Curried Apple and Butternut Squash Soup

The Best Butternut Squash and Apple Curry Soup

A.K.A AUTUMN IN A BOWL

I love fall and everything it brings. Crisp, cooling temperatures, wearing jeans, and bulky sweaters, leaves changing colors, pumpkin patches and the smells of nutmeg and rain to name some favorites. Few things say more about fall than the bounty of produce one can pick up at a local farmers' market including the variety of squash the vendors offer from giant peanut-shaped butternut squash and small green acorn squash to oblong, yellow spaghetti squash and green and orange variegated carnival squash. Because I make every decision based on visuals and impulse, I inevitably come home with at least one of every shape and size - and then realize as I unpack my market bags that I am eating and cooking for one. To relieve myself of any guilt, I plan and make meals I can freeze and eat at a later time, like my favorite harvest soup-using butternut squash. Historically speaking, I have never really been a fan of Butternut squash soup. The texture always reminds me of baby food and the flavor tends to be more like a paste than of my earthy harvest desires, but the addition of apple, carrot, and ginger have completely changed my outlook and now my Fall dreams come true every time I make it.

Ingredients

- 2 tablespoon butter

- 2 tablespoon olive oil

- 1.5 onions chopped

- 2 garlic cloves chopped

- 2 apples peeled and chopped (I used Granny Smith cause of their tartness)

- 1 carrot, chopped

- 2.5 lbs of butternut squash-peeled, seeded and chopped up

- 4 cups chicken broth

- Red pepper flakes

- 2 tablespoons salt + some white pepper

- 1-2 tablespoons yellow curry powder

- 1 teaspoon cinnamon

- Pinch of nutmeg

- 2 tablespoon honey

- 1tablespoon grated fresh ginger

Directions

Put olive oil and butter in a pot & get them warm, adding onions, and garlic. Sauté until they are translucent. Add the apple and carrot & 1/2 curry powder, salt & pep.

Add butternut squash and sauté for about 10 minutes. Add the rest of the spices & honey. When everything is tender, add broth and boil for about 20 minutes. Blend in batches. Additions: Creme fraiche, sour cream, pancetta bits, turkey sausage bits, bacon crumbles or fresh chives. You can make this meal ahead of time and freeze it for later as well

Low Carb Chicken Soup

Low Carb Chicken Soup with Spaghetti Squash Noodles: A veggie-packed low carb soup for that warm and comforting feeling this Fall. Spaghetti squash provides the noodles without all of those pesky carbs!

If you've never heard of Spaghetti Squash, you may be visualizing a heaping plate of pasta with slices of yellow squash mixed in and sprinkled with a generous portion of parmesan cheese. That would be incorrect although we can all agree it sounds delicious! Spaghetti Squash is a vegetable that grows in noodle form and, therefore, lends itself as an excellent substitute for traditional pasta. It holds its own as a side dish but fills the pasta substitute role for those limiting carbohydrates or gluten.

So let's find out more about growing Spaghetti Squash, and how to cook it. Gardeners are a generous bunch, and you might end up with squash and not know what to do with it.

For vegetable gardeners, squash is popular as an easy and fast-growing crop. The Spaghetti Squash variety is no different.

A squash garden requires 8-10 hours of full sun. Once, the danger of frost has, passed, the seeds can be planted directly into the soil. Seedlings emerge a mere 15 days later. Deer do not bother squash plants, but insect activity will need to be monitored.

A ripe gourd is yellow and shaped like a small watermelon. Spaghetti Squash gourds are ready for harvest 70-95 days after seed planting. They can be eaten immediately or stored in a cool place for enjoyment through the fall and winter.

It has a naturally buttery taste so excessive seasoning is not required. It's a good source of Vitamins A, C, Calcium, Iron, Folate, Magnesium, Phosphorus, Potassium and dietary fiber.

Cooking Spaghetti Squash begins with removing the noodles from the gourd. First, the gourd must be baked or microwaved. Then the noodles are separated from the gourd shell by scraping with a fork. The resulting pile of squash noodles is the starting place for many nutritious recipes.

Of course, there are a few more steps necessary to take a large yellow gourd to a pile of spaghetti, but I couldn't include everything here. Once your spaghetti noodles are ready, add ingredients like bacon (what doesn't taste better with bacon?), sausage, cheeses like feta or Parmesan, spinach or onion to make a healthy and tasty dish.

My favorite way of preparing Spaghetti Squash is sautéing in a mixture of olive oil and butter. Soften some diced onions in the oil first; then add the squash. In 10 minutes or so, the dish is ready for the table!

Your family and friends will be very impressed with this wonderful vegetable dish especially if you have grown it yourself.

Low Carb Zuppa Toscana Soup:

You will not miss the potatoes in the comforting low carb Zuppa Toscana soup. Cauliflower makes a nice replacement!

Steps to make Keto Zuppa Toscana Soups

Unlike a traditional Zuppa Toscana soup, you'll like to replace some associated with those high carb components in today's recipe.

Begin by swapping out the taters by using cauliflower. Indeed, you'll know it's not a potato when a person eats it. However Zuppa

Toscana soup is loaded with flavor, and the particular cauliflower absorbs some associated with that flavor while furthermore providing a great alternative for potatoes.

Using a huge soup pot (like this particular dutch oven), brown your sausage and bacon with each other. I chose a moderate Italian sausage (without the particular casings) and a piece of solid sliced bacon. I cut the bacon BEFORE cooking food to assist speed upward the process of cooking food and rendering it simple to put together and eat.

Add within beef bone broth (or beef stock or meat broth) for your cooked chicken and bacon. Why bone tissue broth? I select bone broth because it contains collagen which is GREAT about my joints (remember: CrossFit). This might sound gross, but it essentially tastes the same as beef stock or regular beef broth. You could also use chicken broth, chicken stock, or chicken bone broth instead of the beef flavor. Or vegetable broth for that matter. I found that the beef broth has the richest flavor for today's soup!

Next, add onions, garlic, and cauliflower. For the cauliflower, try to remove as much of the stem as possible, for the best flavor. I used one whole head of organic cauliflower.

Cover your dutch oven and cook for about 15 minutes, until the cauliflower is tender. Add in heavy cream and spinach. Yes, the true Olive Garden Zuppa Toscana Soup recipe contains kale. But you guys, I just don't like the flavor of kale. If you love it, use it. I chose spinach instead because my family LOVES this veggie!

Serve this soup with a sprinkle of Parmesan cheese plus enjoy!

To create this soup, you'll need:

- 1 lb mild Italian sausage

- 4 slices sausage

- 1 head cauliflower

- 32 oz beef bone broth (or beef stock)

- 1 small onion

- 3 cloves garlic

- 1/2 cup weighty whipping cream

- 2 cups fresh spinach (or kale)

- salt and pepper, optional

- crushed red pepper flakes, optional

- shredded parmesan cheese

- Large dutch oven

Beef Stew with Bacon and Mushrooms

This Instant Pot Beef Stew with Bacon and Mushrooms is so full of flavor and so tender! When you use your electric pressure cooker, you can have beef stew in under an hour!

How to Make It

Cook bacon in a heavy 5- to 6-qt. pot over medium heat. Transfer bacon to a large bowl. Pour off all but 1 tbsp. bacon fat from pot, add 1 tbsp. oil, and cook larger sliced mushrooms until beginning to crisp on edges, about 10 minutes; transfer to a second bowl.

Dry beef on paper towels if wet, then season with 1 tsp. salt and the pepper. Add another 1 tbsp. oil to the pot. Brown meat in 3 batches over medium-high heat until nicely browned all over, 20 to 30 minutes total. Add meat to bacon.

Add the remaining 1 tbsp. oil and flour to the pot. Cook over medium heat, stirring often until flour is a shade darker, 2 to 4 minutes. Stir in the remaining 1 1/2 tsp. salt, the thyme, allspice, and tomato paste. Pour in ale and broth; scrape up any browned bits from the bottom of the pot. Add reserved beef and bacon and accumulated juices. Bring to a boil, covered, then reduce heat to maintain a gentle simmer.

Simmer, stirring occasionally, 1 1/2 hours. Meanwhile, peel shallots and separate into lobes. Peel carrots and cut into 1- by 1/2-in. sticks.

Add shallots, cooked and raw mushrooms, potatoes, and carrots to beef and simmer, covered, 1 hour, or until beef is meltingly tender. Sprinkle with chives.

*Find at farmers' markets and well-stocked grocery stores.

TIPS FOR COOKS Shop: Regardless of variety, all mushrooms should smell sweet and earthy and have dry, firm, undamaged caps. If they're spongy or sticky, steer clear. Store: Keep in a document bag (storing them within plastic rots them), perfectly chilled, up to 4 times. Even when they become totally dry, they shall be fine within stews; the juices fat them support. Clean: Clean with a barely wet paper towel. If it could be very dirty or exotic, swish briefly in cool water and scrub along with a tiny brush, then dried out immediately (they get saturated fast). To cook or even not to cook?: Many professionals advise cooking just about all edible mushrooms because, to varying degrees (and according to to the person), they're hard to digest raw. Also, several have toxins that food preparation destroys. However, there's simply no conclusive proof that consuming mild raw mushrooms, specifically in moderation, is dangerous.

Ingredients

• 4 strips thick-cut bacon, cut into 1-in.-wide pieces

• 3 tablespoons vegetable oil, divided

• 2 pounds assorted mushrooms, such as king trumpet, shiitake, and popping*, tough stems trimmed and larger mushrooms thickly sliced

• 2 1/2 pounds beef chuck, cut into 1 1/2-in. pieces

• 2 1/2 teaspoons kosher salt, divided

• 1 teaspoon pepper

• 3 tablespoons whole-wheat flour

• 1 teaspoon dried thyme

• 1/2 teaspoon ground allspice

• 3 tablespoons tomato paste

- 2 bottles (12 oz. each) brown, amber, or bock-style ale, such as Boont Amber Ale

- 1 cup reduced-sodium beef broth

- 8 shallots

- 5 medium carrots

- 1/2-pound baby Yukon Gold potatoes or fingerlings halved lengthwise

- 2 tablespoons snipped fresh chives

TURMERIC BEEF BONE BROTH

Rich, beefy bone broth gets savory upgrades from grass-fed butter (or ghee), seaweed flakes, and anti-inflammatory ground turmeric. Warm your ingredients, and blend for a nutrient-dense and caffeine-free way to perk up.

Turmeric Ginger Bone Broth can be used as the base for a simple soup or used in cooking curries and Asian-flavored stews. To make Turmeric Ginger Pho Bo, pour hot broth over bowls of freshly cooked rice noodles and top with chopped cilantro, torn basil and mint, thinly sliced jalapeños, chopped scallions and paper-thin slices of wild game or beef tenderloin cooked rare. Serve with your favorite hot sauce and wedges of lime.

For Basic Grass-Fed Beef Bone Broth, omit the turmeric, ginger, garlic, cinnamon, star anise, fish sauce, and brown sugar.

Leftover Turmeric Ginger Bone Broth can be kept in the refrigerator for up to 5 days, or stored in the freezer for up to 6 months. Transfer broth into food-grade plastic or glass containers with airtight lids.

Instructions

1. Preheat oven to 400ºF.

2. Rinse and scrub the onion, garlic, ginger, and turmeric. Dry with a kitchen towel and place it on a rimmed baking sheet with the bones. Bake for 1 hour, or until bones and vegetables are deeply browned and caramelized.

3. Place the contents of the pan into a large stockpot, including the crispy browned bits that stick to the pan, and cover with 6 quarts of cold water.

4. Bring to just below a simmer but do not let the contents boil. Adjust the heat until the bubbles are very slowly coming to the surface. As foam forms on the surface of the broth, skim and discard using a fine mesh or slotted spoon. Simmer for 3 hours.

5. As the broth reduces, keep adding water so that the contents of the pot are fully submerged.

6. After 3 hours add the salt, white pepper, cinnamon, and star anise. Continue simmering for another 1 to 2 hours.

7. Add the fish sauce and the brown sugar. Remove from the heat and cool slightly. Taste; adjust for salt, fish sauce, and sugar.

8. Pour the stock over a fine-mesh sieve into a large pot. Discard the solids. Let cool to room temperature and refrigerate for several hours or overnight. Once cold, fat will solidify on the top of the broth. Skim it off and discard.

Ingredients

• 5 lbs marrow bones from grass-fed beef or bison

• 1 large yellow onion unpeeled cut into quarters

• 2 2-inch pieces ginger root unpeeled

• 4 2-inch fingers turmeric root unpeeled, or add 1 teaspoon of turmeric powder to the stockpot.

• 5 cloves garlic unpeeled

• 1 1/2 teaspoon kosher salt

• 1/2 teaspoon ground black pepper

• 1 2-inch piece cinnamon stick

• 2 whole star anise pods

• 1/4 cup fish sauce Shellfish allergy? Use Red Boat brand fish sauce made with anchovies, not shellfish.

• 1 tablespoon brown sugar or use organic coconut sugar

LAMB AND HERB BONE BROTH

Grass-fed lamb is a nourishing protein source — using the bones, you can make a savory and herbaceous broth rich in collagen. To make this keto soup recipe Bulletproof, use pastured bones, skip the roasting, and omit the onion and garlic and use more fresh herbs instead.

How to Make Lamb and Herb Bone Broth?

1. Preheat oven to 200C/390F.

2. Place lamb bones into a roasting pan and cook for 30-40 minutes until well browned.

3. In a large stockpot, add the oil and place over medium heat.

4. Add the onion, carrot, celery, garlic, thyme, and rosemary and saute for 5 minutes.

5. Add the lamb bones and scrape any fat or juices from the roasting pan into the pot.

6. Add 1 gallon of water and allow it to come to a simmer before reducing the heat to low.

7. Simmer for 8-24 hours uncovered, adding more water when the level drops. The amount of water you need will depend on how long you wish to cook the broth.

8. After the broth is cooked for your desired length of time, strain the broth through a fine-mesh strainer.

9. Enjoy hot or chill and use as desired.

Ingredients

• 1-pound lamb bones

- 1 tablespoon olive oil

- 1 small Onion large diced

- 3 medium carrots cut into chunks

- 3 sticks celery roughly chopped

- 3 cloves garlic

- 3 sprigs Rosemary

- 5 sprigs thyme

- 1-3 gallons of water

- Salt optional

What Are The Benefits Of Bone Broth?

Bone broth may help:

- Maintain gut health

- Stave off colds and flu

- Boost the immune system

- Maintain electrolyte levels

- Reduce inflammation

- Protect joints as a good source of collagen

- Keep skin, hair, and nails healthy

We encourage you to use organic lamb when you make lamb bone broth. It is healthier, tastier and contains nothing but pure pasture-fed lamb, not the chemicals and pharmaceuticals that you would find in some mass-produced meat. So, next time you buy some lamb from our Pasture to Plate store, save the bones and make lamb bone broth.

CHICKEN FEET BONE BROTH

Don't be intimidated: Pastured chicken feet create an ultra-gelatinous and nourishing broth packed with collagen and key nutrients. You can even use leftover bone broth as a base in other soups and curries.

Chicken is a "suspect" protein on the Bulletproof Diet because meat (even organic varieties) can come from birds that fed on moldy corn and soy. As a result, chicken has lower-quality fat with more omega-6 fatty acids and potential toxins than other grass-fed animals. If you do eat poultry, look for pastured organic meat (ideally from a local farmer), and only enjoy it a few times per week.

Instructions

1. Set your stock pot on your stove and put 2-4 lbs of chicken feet in pot, if frozen, that is fine... now pour over the chicken feet the apple cider vinegar and let sit (with no flame) for about 45 minutes. This step pulls out all the nutrients from the bones.

2. Now fill the pot with filtered water about 2 inches above the bone and throw in the veggies.

3. Turn to a simmer and put the lid on the pot and let it simmer for 18-24 hours.

4. Turn off and let cool for about an hour, then lift out all the bones/veggies with your Asian strainer into a bowl.

5. Now take another large bowl or a large pot with a lid and put the fine mesh strainer over the top and pour the broth through a strainer to filter out all the grit.

6. Put the lid on or plastic wrap if it is in a bowl and put in the refrigerator to cool down and the fat will separate and rise to the top. I let my cool for about 4 hours or overnight.

7. Take broth out of the fridge and skim off the fat with a large metal spoon. The broth will be like GOOD jelly, which means it is loaded with collagen and gelatin.

8. Set about four or five 1-quart mason jars on the counter and put the wide mouth funnel over one and scoop out the broth with a ladle and put in the jars... Put 3 days' worth of broth in the fridge and freeze the rest. it only stays fresh for about 3-4 days. But you can freeze it for up to one year.

9. IMPORTANT: Only fill mason jars for the freezer 75% full to have room to expand when frozen or the jar will crack! To serve yourself a nice warm mug of bone broth to enjoy, this is what I do: Put 1/2 of the 1 quart mason jar of broth into a saucepan on stove and warm up on medium heat, add 2 scoops of collagen peptides, 1 teaspoon of coconut oil and 1/2 teaspoon of pink Himalayan salt, then pour into a large mug and squeeze 1/4 of a lemon into broth and mix.. ENJOY! I am addicted!

Ingredients

- 2-4 lbs of chicken feet

- 3-4 quarts of filtered water

- 4-8 tablespoons of apple cider vinegar

- 1 onion rough cut

- 4-6 carrots

- 1 celery stalk

BEEF CABBAGE SOUP

Every spoonful of this keto soup recipe contains fall-apart tender chunks of beef, carrots, and cabbage for an unexpectedly filling meal with only 2 net carbs. To make it Bulletproof, use pastured beef and broth, steam your cabbage separately before adding to the soup, and enjoy garlic and onions sparingly.

Ingredients

- 1 pound ground beef

- 2 teaspoons cumin

- 1/2 teaspoon salt

- 1/2 teaspoon ground coriander

- 1 teaspoon garlic powder

- 1/2 teaspoon chili powder (optional)

- 12 ounces diced green chiles

- 1 tablespoon avocado oil

- 1 cup chopped onion

- 6-8 cups chopped cabbage

- 2 cups zucchini, chunks

- 6 cups beef broth

- 1 14 ounces can diced tomatoes

- salt and pepper to taste

Instructions

1. In a large stockpot (add avocado oil if using lean meat) cook ground beef breaking up meat as it's cooking with cumin, salt,

coriander, garlic powder, and chili powder (optional). Once cooked add green chiles.

2. Only drain fat if you have more than 2 tablespoons. Stir in onion, cabbage, and zucchini. Cook until vegetables begin to soften.

3. Add beef broth and simmer for 15-20 minutes. Serve with your favorite toppings.

SLOW COOKER BEEF STEW

With minimal prep time and help from your slow cooker, you can make a rich and hearty stew that pairs perfectly with mashed cauliflower or steamed greens. Every bite gets the flavor from savory herbs and fresh veggies like celery, carrots, and spinach — and every serving is just under 5 net carbs.

Why Slow Cook This Beef Stew?

This slow cooker method is my favorite way to make beef stew because it just allows all that time for the beef to become melt-in-your-mouth tender and also it allows plenty of time for those flavors to meld and marry into utter bliss.

Slow Cooker Beef Stew Ingredients

• Chuck roast

• Olive oil

• Salt and pepper

• Fresh vegetables including yellow onion, celery, garlic, yellow potatoes, and carrots

• Tomato paste

- Low-sodium beef broth or chicken broth

- Worcestershire sauce

- Low-sodium soy sauce

- Fresh herbs including thyme, rosemary, and sage

- Cornstarch

- Frozen peas

How to Make Beef Stew in a Slow Cooker

1. Dab beef dry season with salt and pepper then brown beef in a skillet with olive oil. Transfer to a slow cooker.

2. Saute onions and celery, followed by garlic then tomato paste.

3. Pour in 1 cup of beef broth (to deglaze the pan) along with Worcestershire, soy sauce, thyme, and rosemary.

4. Add potatoes and carrots to slow cooker then pour in beef broth mixture. Pour in remaining broth, season with salt and pepper.

5. Cook on low heat 7 – 8 hours.

6. Whisk cornstarch with water, stir into the stew and cook on high heat an additional 20 minutes to help thicken slightly. Stir in peas and half of the parsley.

7. Serve warm garnished with remaining parsley.

LOW-CARB SLOW-COOKER VEGETABLE BEEF SOUP

This keto soup recipe takes a classic dish to a whole new level with crisp bacon pieces, tender chunks of stew meat, and celery root to replace starchy potatoes. Every bowlful is a miraculous 5 net carbs! Keep it all Bulletproof and use pastured meats and broth, swap red wine vinegar for apple cider vinegar, and skip the garlic and onions. (Since this recipe uses tomato products, also avoid it if you're sensitive to nightshades.)

How to Make Slow Cooker Vegetable Beef Soup:

1. Beef: Place your beef cubes in the slow cooker. You can brown them first or you can skip this step, but with soup recipes, I generally recommend browning the meat as it makes for a better broth! This is optional and won't make a big difference.

2. Vegetables: Add some vegetables and some broth.

3. Cook: Turn it on, and let it cook away until everything is melt in your mouth tender.

4. Can I Make This Vegetable Beef Soup Ahead?

5. Soup is great for making ahead and this easy vegetable beef soup is one of the best because the flavors just get better as it sits.

6. This is a great option for meal prepping on the weekend when you have more spare time, and then simply reheating throughout the week. Because it has no pasta or rice, it can be kept in the refrigerator for up to 4 or 5 days.

Ingredients

- 1 Tablespoon oil

- 1 pound beef cubes

- 1 pound potatoes finely chopped (about 4 medium)

- 2 large carrots peeled and finely chopped

- 2 ribs celery chopped

- 1 small onion finely chopped

- 14 ounces canned diced tomatoes

- 1 1/2 cups chopped green beans fresh or frozen

- 4 cups low sodium beef broth

- 1 cup tomato sauce

- 2 Tablespoons tomato paste

- 2 teaspoons salt

- 2 teaspoons minced garlic

- 1 teaspoon dried parsley

- 1/4 teaspoon paprika

- 1/4 teaspoon black pepper

KETO BEEF SHIRATAKI NOODLE SOUP

With zero-carb shirataki noodles in a warm, beefy broth, this makes the perfect slurpable keto soup recipe. Top with a runny soft-boiled egg, and you can have it all ready in under 30 minutes with just 4.5 net carbs. To stay Bulletproof, use pastured beef and broth, steam bok choy separately (if using) skip the garlic, and use noodles made only from konjac yam (not tofu).

Instructions

1. Boil one egg in a pot.

2. In the meantime, cook meat the way you prefer such as sauteing ground beef with salt and pepper.

3. In another pot, add bone broth and bring to boil. Lower the temperature, add cooked beef meat, garlic, ginger, cardamom, and salt and simmer for 10 minutes.

4. Rinse and drain shirataki noodles and add to the soup. Simmer for another 3 minutes. Add a little bit of sesame oil in for taste (optional). You can also add a few Bok Choy leaves in as well.

5. Divide the soup between 2 bowls, garnish with egg halves and scallions and serve.

Ingredients

For meat

• 5 oz Ground beef (fried minced beef, roast beef, beef meatballs, etc...)

• 1 tbsp olive oil (to saute beef)

• salt and pepper to taste

For Soup & Serving

• 3 cups beef broth (or chicken broth)

• 6 oz shirataki noodles

• 2 garlic cloves minced

• 1 tbsp fresh ginger minced

• 2 scallions sliced

• 1/4 tsp cardamom (optional)

• 1/2 tsp sesame oil optional

- 1 hard-boiled egg halved

- 4 leaves Bok Choy (for serving, optional)

- water (if needed)

- Salt and pepper taste

LOW-CARB PALEO OXTAIL STEW

This keto soup recipe takes a tasty nose-to-tail approach to cooking. Oxtail produces fall-apart tender meat after roasting low and slow in the oven, all in a warm spiced broth with coconut milk and chunky vegetables. Just 10 net carbs for a bowl of savory, meaty flavors.

Instructions

1. Place the oxtail into the slow cooker along with the water and cook on a low heat for 10 hours (the meat should be very tender and fall apart at the end).

2. To make the stew when you're ready to eat, add the tomatoes, garlic, and spices into a saucepan with the oxtail (you can cook it in multiple batches if necessary) and stew for 10-15 minutes.

3. Add salt to taste.

Ingredients

- 4 lb oxtail (chopped into segments – get your butcher to do this if possible)

- 1–2 cups of water (to fill up half the crockpot/slow cooker)

- 2 14oz (400g) cans of diced tomatoes (or 10 fresh tomatoes, diced)

- 10 cloves garlic, crushed

- 4 teaspoons paprika (add more if preferred)

- 2 Tablespoons Italian seasoning (optional – great instead of paprika, e.g., f you don't like any heat in your stew)

- dash of chili powder (optional)

- salt to taste

CREAMY KETO CHICKEN SOUP

No cream here — instead, this keto soup recipe gets a naturally silky texture from fresh pumpkin and coconut cream. With added zest from turmeric, fresh ginger, and lime juice, this comforting chicken soup is just what the doctor ordered.

Ingredients

- 2 tablespoons butter

- 2 cups shredded chicken ~1 large chicken breast

- 4 ounces cream cheese cubed

- 2 tablespoons Stacey Hawkins Garlic Gusto Seasoning

- 14.5 oz chicken broth

- 1/4 cup heavy cream

- salt to taste

- US Customary - Metric

Instructions

1. Melt butter in a saucepan over medium heat.

2. Add shredded chicken to pan and coat with melted butter.

3. As the chicken begins to warm, add cubes of cream cheese and Stacey Hawkins Garlic Gusto seasoning. Mix to blend ingredients.

4. Once the cream cheese has melted and is evenly distributed, add chicken broth and heavy cream. Bring to a boil, then reduce heat to low and simmer for 3-4 minutes.

5. Add salt to taste and serve.

Notes

The garlic gusto seasoning is a combo of mainly parsley, garlic, onion, lemon peel, and paprika.

LOW-CARB, KETO CHICKEN "NOODLE" SOUP

Instead of inflammatory, glutinous wheat noodles, this keto soup recipe uses spiralized daikon radish to create the same slurpable effect. Make this classic more Bulletproof with pastured chicken and chicken stock.

Ingredients

- 2 tablespoons coconut oil

- 1 pound (453 grams) boneless, skinless chicken thighs

- 1 cup diced celery* see note

- 1 cup diced carrots

- ¾ cup (approx. 6) chopped green onion, green part only

- 6 cups chicken stock

- ½ teaspoon dried basil

- ½ teaspoon dried oregano

- 1 teaspoon grey sea salt

- ⅛ teaspoon fresh ground pepper

- 2 cups (300 grams) spiralized daikon noodles* see note

Instructions

1. To make in an Instant Pot: Add coconut oil and chicken thighs to the bowl of your Instant Pot. Set on saute and cook for 10 minutes, until chicken is just about cooked through. Shred with a fork. Add celery, carrots, and onions. Cook for another 2 minutes. Add remaining ingredients. Cover and set on the "soup" setting for 15 minutes. Once complete, add daikon noodles and serve.

2. To make on a stovetop: Add coconut oil and chicken thighs to a large saucepan. Cook on medium for 15 minutes, until chicken, is just about cooked through. Shred with a fork. Add celery, carrots, and onions. Cook for another 5 minutes. Add remaining ingredients. Cover and bring to a boil. Reduce heat and simmer for 25 minutes. Once complete, add daikon noodles and serve.

Notes

Celery: If you're severely FODMAP sensitive, you can replace the celery with more carrots, or use radishes!

Daikon Noodles: You can find daikon in your local grocery store. I was able to find some at health food stores, Superstore, and Walmart carried it, too. Best if made into keto noodles with a spiralizer, but a vegetable peeler will work as well.

CHICKEN KETO RAMEN

This soup recipe uses one of the easiest keto noodle replacements available — shredded cabbage! Add it to a gingery broth with runny ramen eggs for a warming meal with just 4.4 net carbs.

Ingredients

- 1 small organic chicken about 3lbs
- 12 cups water
- 2 organic chicken broth cubes we use organic cubes or powder that are ALSO free of hydrogenated oils.
- 4 large eggs
- 2 tbsp salt
- 2 packs shirataki noodles about 1 lb in total
- 6 green onions chopped
- 4 tbsp Gluten-free soy sauce

Instructions

1. In a large pot, bring your water to a boil and add your chicken to it. Lower, the heat to medium-low, add your chicken stock cubes and salt. Cover and cook for 1 hour and 15 minutes.

2. Remove your chicken from the pot, leave your broth uncovered and let it simmer for another 45 minutes on low heat. Once your broth is ready, pass through a strainer to get rid of any impurities.

3. Once your chicken has cooled down, strip the carcass of all its meat and place it in a bowl.

4. In a medium pot, bring 4 cups of water to a boil and carefully place your 4 eggs in there. Cook for exactly 6 minutes for perfectly runny egg yolks.

It's Ramen Bowl Building Time

1. For each bowl, place half a pack of shirataki noodles, one tbsp of soy sauce, as much chicken as you like, one soft boiled egg cut in half of the course and a handful of chopped green onions.

2. Serve & Enjoy!

Notes

Please keep in mind that while this recipe is crafted for 4 bowls of ramen, the broth itself is not. As a result, you will have lots of leftover chicken broth (another 4-5 bowls). I made this to have ramen broth for the entire week.

CHICKEN CAULIFLOWER RICE SOUP

If you miss chicken and rice soup, try this keto soup recipe. With tender pearls of riced cauliflower and a creamy broth, you won't miss the grains. Make this soup Bulletproof with pastured meat and broth, skip the onion, use grass-fed ghee, and steam your cauliflower rice separately before adding to the pot.

Ingredients

- 2 medium chicken breasts
- 2 cups celery, diced
- 1 cup carrots, diced
- 6 cups vegetable broth

- 3 cups cauliflower, uncooked and riced

- 3 bay leaves

- ½ t turmeric

- Salt and pepper, to taste

Instructions

1. Turn the crockpot on high and allow it to preheat while you chop the veggies.

2. To the crockpot, add chicken breasts, celery, vegetable broth, bay leaves, turmeric, salt, and pepper.

3. Leave crockpot set on high to cook 6 hours.

4. Check crockpot at 6 hours to see if the chicken is cooked. It should be tender and you should be able to pull it apart easily with a spatula or spoon. If not, allow cooking for another hour until you can shred the chicken.

5. After chicken is cooked, reduce crockpot to low. Add cauliflower rice. Cook another 20 minutes to cook the cauliflower rice until tender.

6. Transfer to a bowl and serve immediately.

CHICKEN AVOCADO LIME SOUP

This low-carb take on tortilla soup gets the zesty flavor from jalapeños, cumin, and lime juice, all mixed with creamy avocado chunks and tender pieces of chicken. Each bowlful is only 8 net carbs. To make this keto soup recipe Bulletproof, use pastured chicken and broth, skip the garlic, avoid tomatoes if you're sensitive to nightshades, and omit the garnishes.

Ingredients

- 1 1/2 lbs boneless skinless chicken breasts*

- 1 Tbsp olive oil

- 1 cup chopped green onions (including whites, mince the whites)

- 2 jalapeños, seeded and minced (leave seeds if you want soup spicy, omit if you don't like heat)

- 2 cloves garlic, minced

- 4 (14.5 oz) cans low-sodium chicken broth

- 2 Roma tomatoes, seeded and diced

- 1/2 tsp ground cumin

- Salt and freshly ground black pepper

- 1/3 cup chopped cilantro

- 3 Tbsp fresh lime juice

- 3 medium avocados, peeled, cored and diced

- Tortilla chips, Monterrey jack cheese, sour cream for serving (optional)

Instructions

1. In a large pot heat 1 Tbsp olive oil over medium heat. Once hot, add green onions and jalapenos and saute until tender, about 2 minutes, adding garlic during the last 30 seconds of sauteing.

2. Add chicken broth, tomatoes, cumin, season with salt and pepper to taste and add chicken breasts. Bring mixture to a boil over medium-high heat.

3. Then reduce heat to medium, cover with a lid and allow to cook, stirring occasionally, until chicken has cooked through 10 - 15 minutes (cook time will vary based on the thickness of chicken breasts).

4. Reduce burner to warm heat, remove chicken from pan and let rest on a cutting board 5 minutes, then shred chicken and return to soup. Stir in cilantro and lime juice.

5. Add avocados to soup just before serving (if you don't plan on serving the soup right away, I would recommend adding the avocados to each bowl individually, about 1/2 an avocado per serving). Serve with tortilla chips, cheese, and sour cream if desired.

6. *For thicker chicken breasts, cut breasts in half through the length (thickness) of the breasts, they will cook faster and more evenly.

30-MINUTE TURMERIC CHICKEN SOUP

Earthy turmeric pairs perfectly with chicken and hearty vegetables in this keto soup recipe. To cut down on carbs, use vegetables like cauliflower and chard (steamed before adding to the soup). For a Bulletproof take on this soup, use pastured meats and broth and full-fat canned coconut milk.

Ingredients

- 2 and 1/2 tsp turmeric powder (like this)

- 1 and 1/2 tsp cumin powder (like this)

- 1/8 tsp cayenne powder (like this)

- 3 small boneless chicken thighs

- 2 tbsp coconut oil, ghee, or butter – divided

- 1 small onion, diced

- 4 cups of chopped vegetables (I used carrots, cauliflower, and broccoli)

- 4 cups good quality broth (bone broth OR vegetable broth)

- 1 cup of water

- 1 bay leaf

- 1 tsp grated fresh ginger

- 2 cups chard, de-stemmed, and sliced into thin ribbons

- 1/2 cup full-fat coconut milk (or any milk of choice)

GARNISH

- fresh cilantro

- lemon wedges

- red pepper flakes

Instructions

1. Mix turmeric, cumin, and cayenne in a small bowl and set aside.

2. Chop chicken thighs into small bite-size pieces (I use kitchen shears for this) and set aside.

3. Melt 1 tbsp of fat of choice in a medium soup pot. Add onions and cook until translucent, about 3 minutes. Add half of the turmeric spice mixture and the 4 cups of vegetables and cook for another 3-4 minutes.

4. Add broth, water, bay leaf, and ginger to the pot and bring to a boil. Lower heat and simmer until vegetables are fork-tender, about 8-10 minutes. Turn off heat and stir in coconut milk and greens, allowing the heat to wilt the greens.

5. While vegetables are cooking, heat remaining one tablespoon of fat in a large skillet. Add chopped chicken pieces and cook until no longer pink on the outside, about 5 minutes. Add remaining turmeric spice mix and cook until chicken is thoroughly cooked inside, about another 5 minutes.

6. Once vegetables are done, ladle soup into your favorite bowls, top with cooked chicken and garnish with fresh cilantro, red pepper flakes, and a squeeze of lemon.

PALEO KETO LOW-CARB CHICKEN NOODLE SOUP

This take on chicken noodle soup uses classic ingredients like carrot and celery, plus spaghetti squash "noodles" as a gluten-free and keto swap. Even though the squash takes time to cook, you only need 10 minutes to prep for a filling soup with only 3 net carbs. Make this keto soup recipe more Bulletproof with pastured chicken and broth — plus, skip the onion, or enjoy only on occasion.

Ingredients

• 2 tablespoon ghee

- 1 cup small diced onion

- 1 cup small-diced celery

- ½ cup small diced carrots

- 2 cloves garlic minced

- 2 bay leaves

- 2 tablespoons apple cider vinegar

- 1-pound boneless skinless chicken thighs, diced

- 1 teaspoon fine salt

- 1 teaspoon garam masala, I use this one, it's nightshade-free

- 1 teaspoon turmeric

- 1 teaspoon cumin

- 1 teaspoon onion powder

- 1 cup pumpkin purée

- 3 cups Bonafide Provisions chicken bone broth

- 2 bags Thrive Market shirataki noodles or Miracle Noodles

- 3 slices crispy bacon for garnish

Instructions

1. Heat your pressure cooker on sauté mode. Add in ghee and veggies and sauté with bay leaves until tender, about 5 minutes.

2. Deglaze with vinegar, then add in seasonings and chicken and sauté, stirring often until browned. About 5 minutes.

3. Mix in the pumpkin and the bone broth. Cancel the sauté function on your pressure cooker and set to cook on high for

20 minutes. Manually release pressure, open the lid and stir in the noodles.

4. Garnish with bacon bits, fresh herbs (like sage) or chopped nuts!

5. To make it AIP compliant: omit the garam masala, and cumin, add in ½ teaspoon ground ginger, ½ teaspoon ground cinnamon, 1 teaspoon garlic powder

Chicken Zoodle Soup:

Everybody's favorite soup gets a low-carb makeover that maintains its classic taste.

Cold weather brings on sickness especially if you have school-age children. When fall approaches, commonly, I will get a cold since school starts at the end of summer and goes into fall. My throat becomes irritated, and the nose begins to run. Since it's that time of year, you want to try to fight off any illness before it takes hold of you, and the best way I have found is to start eating plenty of soup.

Eating hot soup and drinking hot herbal tea is one of my go-to meals for sickness. A hot bowl of chunky chicken noodle soup is the best medicine. What or why would a child turn down chicken noodle soup? Sometimes my child might get set in her ways and put up a fight but once she tastes it then her mind changes quickly.

Chicken noodle soup is the easiest recipe to make. I make mine simple since I am only concerned with the hot liquid. The chicken, noodles, and vegetables are a bonus. If you ever have a sore throat and it hurts to swallow, I suggest sipping on broths and hot tea until your throat feels better. I am sharing with you a simple chicken noodle soup I make at home when I feel under the weather.

Ingredients

- 1 lb chicken breast/chicken tenders

- 1 onion

- 2 to 3 stalks celery

- 2 to 3 carrots

- 1 Tsp chicken seasoning

- 1 Tsp thyme

- 2 bay leaves

- ½ package of egg noodles

- Salt and pepper to taste

I wash the chicken then I cover with water in a saucepan and start cooking the chicken. I like to cook the chicken a bit before cutting it into chunks. Season the water generously with salt and pepper, chicken seasoning, and add 2 bay leaves. I chop the onion, celery, and carrot. In a skillet, I sauté the onion and celery until tender. Before the chicken cooks thoroughly, I strain the chicken liquid through a sieve. I remove the chicken and place it on a cutting board then cut into pieces to finishing cooking. I add the meat back to the sieved liquid then add the vegetables and noodles. If you already have cooked chicken and chicken broth then you can add the chicken to the broth along with the vegetables and cook until vegetables are tender. Cook the soup until vegetables are tender and the noodles al dente. Serve with some crackers or a grilled cheese sandwich on the side.

Instant Pot Loaded Cauliflower Soup:

Who needs spuds? Cauliflower is plenty comforting when loaded up with bacon goodness.

Now that the weather is getting cooler it's soup season and last weekend, I made a big batch of this awesome Instant Pot Loaded Cauliflower Soup in my pressure cooker. It is rich, creamy, and topped with some of my favorite things...cheese, bacon, and sour cream!!

In the pressure cooker this creamy cauliflower soup only has to cook on high for 10 minutes, then a quick puree with an immersion blender and it's ready to serve.

How to Make Cauliflower Soup in the Instant Pot:

1. Place the cauliflower, onion, and chicken broth in the pot of your Instant Pot and then lock the lid in place. Turn the top valve to "Sealing."

2. Press "Manual," then press "Pressure" until the light on "High Pressure" lights up, then adjust the +/- buttons until the timer reads 10 minutes.

3. When the time is up press "Cancel" to stop the cooking and then wait 10 minutes as the Instant Pot does a natural release. After 10 minutes carefully, turn the vent to "Venting" to release the remaining steam.

4. Remove the lid and add the lemon juice then use an immersion blender to puree the soup until it is smooth and creamy.

5. Add salt and pepper to taste.

6. Ladle the cauliflower soup into bowls and top with bacon, chives, sour cream, and cheddar cheese.

Can I Freeze Cauliflower Soup?

Yes! I suggest portioning the cauliflower soup out into individual servings so you can heat smaller amounts as needed. To freeze let the soup cool completely and then portion into small airtight containers and freeze.

When you are ready to reheat, you can place the frozen soup in a microwave-safe bowl and microwave for 2-3 minutes or until heated through.

If you prefer to use the stovetop, you can place the frozen soup in a small saucepan on the stove and heave over medium heat, stirring often, until it is heated through.

Ingredients

- 50 ounces Cauliflower, roughly chopped

- 4 ounces Onion roughly chopped

- 4 cups Chicken broth

- 2 tablespoons Lemon juice

- Salt & pepper to taste

- 10 slices Bacon

- 2 tablespoons Chives

- 10 tablespoons Sour Cream

- 10 ounces Cheddar cheese

Instructions

1. Place the cauliflower, onion, and chicken broth in the pot of your Instant Pot and then lock the lid in place. Turn the top valve to "Sealing."

2. Press "Manual," then press "Pressure" until the light on "High Pressure" lights up, then adjust the +/- buttons until the timer reads 10 minutes.

3. When the time is up press "Cancel" to stop the cooking and then wait 10 minutes as the Instant Pot does a natural release. After 10 minutes carefully, turn the vent to "Venting" to release the remaining steam.

4. Remove the lid and add the lemon juice then use an immersion blender to puree the soup until it is smooth and creamy.

5. Add salt and pepper to taste.

6. Ladle the cauliflower soup into bowls and top with bacon, chives, sour cream, and cheddar cheese.

Notes

5 net carbs

Keto Bacon Cheeseburger Soup:

This blend of beef, cheddar, and Worcestershire tastes so much like a cheeseburger, you won't miss the bun at all.

When I'm not working on my many businesses, I'm in the kitchen, cooking' up to something' good! My husband is like a big old' kid, he is very picky when it comes to food. So, I like to throw together my little recipes using ingredients I know he loves. Also, I get bored eating the same things, so I have to change it up now and then. So, one day, I thought, "Why do burgers have to be made into patties? Why don't I just mix all the ingredients, and throw it on a hoagie roll?" So, that's what I did... And OMG! I can't believe how great of an idea that was! It's all the same ingredients as a regular hamburger, but the flavor is soooooo different! And delicious! This is now my husband's favorite meal! If I had kids, I'm sure it would be their favorite, too! Just cook up the ingredients, and dress it as you would a normal hamburger. I guarantee the whole family will absolutely love it, and beg for it often. It's also fairly quick to make, which is good for our work at home wives whose work never seems to end. Enough with the suspense, already! Here's the recipe...

Ingredients:

- 1 lb Hamburger Meat
- 1 Pack of Bacon
- Medium Block of Velveeta Cheese (Cubed)
- 1 Medium Onion (Diced, optional)
- 1 TBS Garlic Salt
- 1 TBS Tony Chachere's
- 1 tsp Salt (optional)
- 1/4 C Milk
- Butter
- Philly Cheesesteak Hoagie Rolls

Directions:

1. First, Grab a large non-stick pot, and pre-heat it over medium-high heat. While it's heating, stack your bacon on a cutting board, and cut it into small squares.

2. Next, throw your bacon, and onions if you desire, into the heated pot, and cook until it's almost crispy, or crispy if you like it that way.

3. Once your bacon is cooked, add the pound of hamburger meat to the mixture. Sprinkle garlic salt, Tony's, and salt over the mixture. Cook until meat is browned.

4. Drain grease from the mixture.

5. Next, add milk, and cheese to the mixture. Over medium-low heat, stir until cheese has completely melted.

6. Now, butter your hoagie rolls, and grill over medium-high heat until golden brown.

7. Place mixture on a grilled roll, and dress with your favorite toppings. (Lettuce, tomato, mayo, mustard, ketchup, etc.)

There it is! So, cheesy and so delicious! I'm sure it will become a new favorite at your house, just like it is at mine.

Instant Pot Broccoli Cheese Soup:

This Broccoli Cheese Soup is ready in under 30 minutes! I use cheese as the thickener instead of flour. I also give tips to keep the cheese from not melting and sinking to the bottom of the pot.

Butter, cheese, and vegetables — a keto dieter's trusty starter pack — make a mean soup.

Broccoli, an ancient food that existed during the Roman Empire, is something we still enjoy today. It has been around for centuries, made its way to Europe and then was finally introduced to the North American diet around 300 years ago.

Why broccoli?

If you are trying to stay healthy, lean and strong this is the food for you. This amazing food is considered to have a low sugar load which means it will not spike your blood sugar level. Foods that fit into this category help you to lose weight naturally.

One of the best reasons to eat broccoli is for the isothiocyanates it contains. Isothiocyanates are a type of phytonutrient known to prevent cancer and to help fight against cancer.

Fiber aids our body in the elimination process and helps us to maintain optimal health. Broccoli is an excellent source of dietary fiber. If your diet is high in meat, dairy and eggs adding broccoli can provide you with fiber, nutrients, minerals, vitamins and just some lovely color for your dinner plate.

This incredible food can help you reach your optimal health and optimal maintainable weight. It is loaded with vitamins and contains more vitamins than the average orange. These are some of the nutrients that you will find in broccoli:

• Vitamins A, B6, C and E

• Calcium, Magnesium, Zinc, Copper, Manganese, and Selenium

• Choline, Folate

How can I add broccoli to my healthy balanced meals?

Raw or frozen broccoli is available in almost any grocery store. Whenever possible, I recommend purchasing it raw. Processed foods, even frozen products, contain higher levels of sodium than the food would naturally have. Part of the process of freezing fruits and vegetables is the destruction of the enzymes in the food. The fruits and vegetables that we eat have natural enzymes in them. These substances help our body in many ways including digestion. If we start raw, we have a better chance of receiving the full benefit of the food we are eating.

Broccoli is a very versatile food. It can be eaten raw, cooked, in soups and stews, in quiche and omelets, on platters, as a side dish for the main course, as a snack, as part of a salad or as the main ingredient of the salad. One of the reasons I like broccoli is its vibrant green color. It can instantly make the appearance of any meal fun and exciting. If you like to "play" with your food, try cutting broccoli into little green florets and arranging those next to slices of tomatoes or cucumber. This will add a quick and decorative touch to any meal. Another great feature is that you can decide on how big or small you want the florets allowing you to fit broccoli into any meal idea.

Broccoli can easily be overcooked and when it is, it turns mushy and the vibrant green color disappears. Try steaming this delicate vegetable. Cut the florets into the desired size and place them in a steamer with a little water in the bottom. The florets should not sit in the water. When the water reaches a full boil, turn off the element, remove the pot from the stovetop and let it sit. The heat from the water will cook the broccoli, the florets will not be mushy and the color will be vibrant.

The stems and the florets are both edible and have slightly different flavors. Try them both raw and cooked. You may find you have a preference. You might like the stems raw and the florets cooked or the stems cooked and the florets raw. Whichever way you prefer, slip a little broccoli into your healthy balanced meals.

Ten Ways to Include Broccoli into Your Everyday Meals

1. In Salads

Traditionally, we tend to think of salads like lettuce, tomatoes, and cucumbers. You can create variety to this type of salad by simply adding some broccoli florets.

Cooked salads made with pasta, potatoes or shrimp look lovely with broccoli florets. You can add cooked or raw florets depending on the texture you desire. Cook florets gently to maintain some of the crispness and to prevent them from being damaged when mixed into the salad.

2. As the Main Ingredient of a Salad

Making a salad with broccoli as the main ingredient is easy to do. You can use it raw or gently steam it. The salad dressing that you use will help you decide what to add to the salad. Try to be colorful in your food choices. You could add tomatoes pieces or walnuts. An appealing appearance is half the battle in making food taste good.

3. Veggie Platters and Salad Plates

Veggie platters are easy to make and there are no set rules regarding what to add. Broccoli makes a great division between red peppers and tomatoes on a vegetable platter. Be creative by mixing colors, shapes, and textures.

Children love to be entertained and fun food is a great place to start. Add variety to their meals by creating a salad plate in shape of a face. Small broccoli florets for hair, cucumber slices for eyes, a cherry tomato for a nose and almonds in the shape of a mouth. Or if you would rather do a landscape; broccoli florets can double as trees in the background. Be creative and "play" with your food.

4. As Sprouts

Some children (and adults too) have decided that they do not like broccoli - which is very unfortunate. But there is a solution!

Broccoli sprouts, similar to alfalfa sprouts in appearance, are an excellent substitute. These young, small greens have a bit of zest to them. They are great on sandwiches or with brown rice crackers and tahini spread. Try replacing the broccoli florets in your child's salad (described above) with sprouts to create a wild hairstyle.

5. With Eggs

Scrambled eggs, omelets, and quiche are enhanced with the addition of bright green broccoli florets. For softer florets, you may have to steam them slightly. Since eggs and dairy products lack fiber adding broccoli not only makes the meal interesting by adding color but also adds fiber.

6. In Soups

Regardless of the base of your soup, broccoli can be added to almost any mixed vegetable soup, even borscht. It can be chopped into small pieces, blended to make cream soups or left as larger decorative pieces. Next time you make home-made chicken soup, add some lovely green florets and enjoy the color combinations.

7. As a Side Dish

Broccoli as a side dish can brighten up a meal. It can be served with a cheese or cream sauce, or you can drizzle some heart-healthy olive oil with seasonings and herbs over top.

8. In Salsa, Pesto, and Stir-fry

There are so many ways to combine broccoli with your meals. Consider chopping it into fine pieces and adding them to your salsa or pesto. Large broccoli florets can turn the appearance of a stir fry around. Add some large florets when the stir fry is almost ready. The broccoli only needs a few minutes to steam from the heat and juices of the stir fry. Just placing it on top and covering it for a few minutes should be enough to cook the broccoli and maintain the color.

9. For a Snack

Broccoli is great as a snack because it does not cause blood sugar levels to snack. If you do not have it planned as part of your healthy balanced meals for the day, you can add broccoli in as s snack. Cutting broccoli stems into long strips makes it easy to pack for a snack. Try adding a little cashew or almond butter for a yummy healthy treat. Children will enjoy dipping the strips into the nut butter.

10. A Garnish

Garnishes are usually thought of as pieces of herbs such as cilantro or parsley, a piece of lettuce or a slice of citrus. Consider broccoli as a garnish. It can be very decorative and its shape allows you to be creative with it. Cut into slices, the pale green of the stem adds a nice touch beside carrot strips and is a great replacement for celery, the small florets can be used to decorate and add color to any plain colored meal, and finely chopped or minced broccoli looks lovely as a garnish on a bowl of cream soup.

Conclusion

Sprouts, strips, florets, and garnishes are all great ways to include broccoli into your healthy balanced meals and healthy snacks. Be creative and enjoy the health benefits of broccoli.

Low-Carb Buffalo Chicken Soup with Blue Cheese:

This wholesome dish reimagines the beloved chicken-wing app into one warming bowl. This Keto Buffalo Chicken soup recipe isn't like eating a liquified buffalo wing if that's what you're thinking. The flavors are a lot more subtle than that but very noticeable. It's creamy and satisfying, all while hitting your low carb high fat keto macros – so no guilt!

As a bonus, this Keto Buffalo Chicken Soup is very easy to make – and works perfectly with some shredded rotisserie chicken meat, so you can get away with very little cooking to get dinner on the table!

If you haven't tried it yet, I highly recommend putting this Keto chicken soup on your list ASAP! It's guaranteed to be a hit with the entire family!

Ingredients

- 1 lb chicken breast, cubed

- 32 oz chicken stock

- 1/2 cup buffalo wing sauce

- 4 green onions, chopped

- 2 medium carrots, chopped

- 2 ribs celery, diced

- 2 cloves garlic, minced

- 1 cup sharp cheddar cheese, shredded

- 2/3 cup Parmesan cheese, shredded

- 1/4 cup blue cheese crumbles, extra for garnish if desired

- 2 tbsp Italian flat-leaf parsley, chopped (optional for garnish)

Instructions

1. Heat slow cooker on a low setting.

2. To the slow cooker, add chicken, chicken stock, buffalo wing sauce, green onion, carrots, celery, and garlic. Cover and cook 6 hours.

3. Add cheddar, parmesan, and blue cheeses. Stir until cheeses are melted and mixed in. Cover and cook 1 additional hour.

4. Garnish with blue cheese crumbles and parsley before serving.

Roasted Poblano Chicken Cauliflower Soup:

Elevate plain old' cauliflower soup with tender shredded chicken and smoky roasted poblano peppers.

Here's how you make it...

Preheat your oven to 350°F. Cut 2 heads of cauliflower into florets of roughly the same size. You want them to be around the same size so that they cook evenly in the oven. Place the cauliflower in a single layer on an aluminum-foiled lined baking sheet. Drizzle some oil (olive or canola will work just fine) over the cauliflower, somewhere around 3 tablespoons. Then season generously with Kosher Salt and Freshly Ground Black Pepper. Take your hands and move the cauliflower all around to evenly coat the florets with the oil, salt, and pepper.

Pop the baking sheet in the oven for about 25 – 30 minutes, stirring the cauliflower halfway through. When the cauliflower is done, it will be fork-tender and have some spots of golden-brown. Kind of like this:

Roasting the cauliflower, as with all vegetables, brings out and concentrates its natural sugars. The cauliflower slightly caramelizes during the process, transforming it into something so much better than just, well, cauliflower. This roasting "trick" works with all vegetables by the way... it's my favorite way to eat vegetables.

At this point, scrape the cauliflower into a saucepot and add around 4 cups of chicken stock. You can make your own, which is time-consuming but super easy and delicious (recipe for that at the bottom of this post) or you can use store-bought chicken or vegetable stock. Buying stock is the easier route to go, but make sure to buy quality. I typically use Trader Joe's brand, but I've heard that Cooks Illustrated is partial to Swanson.

Bring the cauliflower-stock mixture to a boil over medium-high heat, then lower to a simmer and let it go for about 15-20 minutes. Let cool, then transfer cauliflower to a blender with a slotted spoon. Add in just a couple cups of the stock and purée. Add in more stock as you see fit until it reaches a thick soup consistency. You might use all the stock, you might not, depending on how thick you want the soup to be.

Pour the soup through a fine-mesh sieve placed on top of a large bowl. Stir the soup through the fine-mesh sieve and discard any solids left behind.

*If you aren't planning on serving the soup right away, you can refrigerate the cauliflower soup mixture at this point for a day or two until ready to serve.

The last step is an easy one: pour the cauliflower mixture into a pot and bring to a simmer over medium-low heat. Stir in about 3/4 cup of heavy cream and 2 puréed poblano chiles (keep reading for how to make that). Season with salt and pepper heat until warmed through.

Let's take a side step here for that poblano purée and also to make the pepper relish garnish (try to say that 5 times fast) …

When the cauliflower was done roasting in the oven, crank up the heat to 375°F. It's time to roast 3 poblano chiles and 1 red bell pepper. The same process as the cauliflower: put the peppers on an aluminum-lined baking sheet and drizzle with a tablespoon or two of canola oil and sprinkle with Kosher salt and pepper. Use your hand and toss the peppers to evenly coat with the oil. (In the picture below, there are more peppers than you need for this recipe... I was roasting up some additional ones for some other eats).

Put the tray of peppers into the oven. Check on your roasting peppers now and again, rotating/turning the peppers with tongs about every 6-8 minutes or until the cooked side has blistered with some brown char marks. The poblanos are normally smaller than red bell peppers, so they may be done first. Typically, it takes around 20 – 30 minutes depending upon the size of your peppers. They will have brown char marks and wrinkled skin when they are done, kind of like this:

Place your peppers in a bowl and cover with plastic wrap for at least 10 minutes. This process will create steam, making the skins easier to peel.

After the 10 minutes (or longer) has passed, peel the skin off the peppers with your fingers and remove the seeds from inside the peppers. The skins should slide right off, but you may have some stubborn spots here and there. ***You might want to wear gloves when peeling and handling these poblano chiles. They can leave your hands (and anywhere your hand touches) with a burning sensation.

Once you are done peeling and seeding, finely chop 1 poblano pepper, and the 1 red bell pepper. With the other 2 poblanos, place into a food processor or blender and puree:

So, remember the puréed poblanos = soup / the finely chopped poblano and red pepper = part of the garnish. Okay, it's plating time!

Fill bowls with your soup. I like to garnish mine with a couple of cilantro leaves and a "pepper relish" of sorts. Here's how you make it: Take that finely chopped roasted red bell pepper and poblano chile and place them in a bowl. Hit it with a splash of red wine or sherry vinegar and a squeeze of honey (equal parts honey/vinegar, somewhere around 1 tsp – 1 TBL each). Throw in a pinch of Kosher salt and Freshly Ground Black Pepper. Taste and adjust the honey/vinegar/salt/pepper as necessary. This "relish" adds beautiful color to the soup and also brings an added depth of flavor.

Serve some blue corn chips on the side with softened fresh goat cheese. The tangy-ness of the goat cheese goes well with the richness of this soup.

Ingredients

- 2 heads cauliflower, cut into florets

- 4 tablespoons olive or canola oil

- 4 cups Chicken Stock (see recipe below or buy quality low-sodium chicken broth or vegetable broth)

- 3/4 cup heavy cream

- 3 poblano chiles

- 1 red bell pepper

- Blue Corn Tortilla Chips

- Fresh Goat Cheese

- Cilantro, roughly chopped

- Splash of Red Wine Vinegar or Sherry Vinegar

- Squeeze of Honey

- Kosher Salt and Freshly Ground Black Pepper

Instructions

1. Preheat the oven to 350°F. Put the cauliflower on a large baking sheet covered in aluminum foil. Drizzle with approximately 3 tablespoons of the oil, season with Kosher salt and freshly ground black pepper, and toss to coat. Place the cauliflower into the oven and roast, stirring the cauliflower around a bit halfway through the process, until the cauliflower starts to turn golden brown and is soft, about 25 – 30 minutes.

2. Raise the heat of the oven to 375°F. Place the 3 poblano chiles and 1 red bell pepper on a baking sheet covered in aluminum foil. Drizzle with approximately 1 tablespoon of oil, season with Kosher salt and freshly ground black pepper. Toss to coat. Place, the tray of peppers into the oven and roast for about 20-30 minutes, turning/rotating with tongs about every 6-8 minutes, until the peppers, are blistered with brown char marks and the skins are wrinkled. Remove from the oven and place the peppers in a bowl, cover with plastic wrap, and let sit for at least 10 minutes. This will allow the skins to loosen. Remove skins and seeds from the chiles and pepper.

3. Place 2 of the roasted poblano chiles into a blender or food processor and purée. Finely chop the other roasted poblano chile and roasted red bell pepper.

4. While the peppers are roasting, scrape the cauliflower into a medium saucepan and add the stock. Bring to a boil over medium-high heat, then lower the heat and simmer for 15-20 minutes.

5. Let cool a bit and then ladle all of the cauliflower with a slotted spoon from the saucepan into a blender. Add a couple of cups of the stock. Puree until smooth, adding more of the stock from the saucepan until you reach a thick soup consistency. You may use all the stock, you may not, depending on how much cauliflower you have and how thick/thin you want your soup to be. Strain the soup through a fine-mesh sieve into a clean pot. The soup can be made up to this point a couple of days in advance. Store in a covered bowl in the refrigerator.

6. When ready to serve, bring the mixture to a gentle simmer over medium heat and whisk in the heavy cream and poblano puree. Season with Kosher Salt and Freshly Ground Black Pepper. Cook for about 5 minutes, or until just warmed through.

7. Meanwhile, prepare the "pepper relish" garnish. Combine the finely chopped roasted poblano chile and red bell pepper with a splash of red wine or sherry vinegar and a squeeze of honey. The vinegar and honey should be approximately equal parts. Season with salt and pepper. Taste and adjust seasonings to your liking. This can be made a day or two ahead of time.

8. Serve soup in bowls topped with a little of the pepper relish and a little chopped cilantro. Serve alongside tortilla chips topped with softened goat cheese.

Instant Pot Chili Verde:

Spice up a dreary day with zesty tomatillos and jalapeños. Instant Pot Chile Verde is everything you dreamed of in classic Chile Verde, in a fraction of the usual cooking time! If you've stayed away from making Chile Verde at home because you don't have 8 hours to tend the slow cooker, this recipe is for you! Tender, fall-apart pork is the center of this Instant Pot Chile Verde recipe.

Ingredients

• 3-3.5 lbs pork loin sirloin roast, or pork shoulder, trimmed of fat and cut into one-inch pieces

• 1 tablespoon of sea salt

• 1 teaspoon pepper

• 3 tablespoons olive oil

• juice of one lime

• 1/4 cup flour

• 1 onion white, yellow or sweet, chopped (about 1 1/2 cups)

• 2-3 cloves garlic chopped

• 7 Anaheim peppers (about 3 cups chopped) or 3- 7 oz cans green chiles

• 1-2 jalapeños

• 5-6 tomatillos a little larger than golf ball size husked

• 1 cup chicken beef or vegetable broth

• avocado tortillas for serving

Instructions

1. Place rack on second to the top level of the oven and turn the oven to broil.

2. Lightly spray a jelly roll pan with cooking oil. Wash the Anaheim peppers, jalapeño, and tomatillos. Slice in half and remove stems. Seed the jalapeño and Anaheim's and discard the seeds if you do not want the Chile Verde to be spicy. Do not seed the tomatillos.

3. Place the Anaheim peppers, Jalapeño and tomatillos on the baking sheet cut side down. Broil for about 7-10 minutes or until browned. Remove and let cool.

4. Chop the onion and garlic.

5. Chop the boiled veggies and set aside with the onion and garlic.

6. Place the Instant Pot on a sturdy surface where the pot can vent steam, away from under cabinets.

7. Turn the Instant Pot to the Sauté mode and let heat up.

8. When the Instant Pot is heated up, pour the oil into the pot. Brown, the meat in two batches, removing the first batch to a plate after browning. While the meat is cooking, season with salt and pepper.

9. After, the second batch of meat is browned, add the first batch of browned meat back to the pan. Squeeze the lime juice over all of the meat and mix with a large spoon. Sprinkle the flour over the meat in the pan and continue cooking until all of the flour disappears and the meat is coated with flour. Cook for about 2-3 minutes on high. Do not place the lid on the pan yet.

10. Dump all of the chopped peppers, onion and garlic into the Instant Pot with the meat mixture.

11. Pour in broth.

12. Make sure the pressure release valve is turned to the "seal" position and the sealing ring is properly placed inside of the lid. Place the lid on the pot and turn the lid to the closed position.

13. Push the "meat/stew" button, or hit "manual" and use the + button to add 35 minutes to the timer. Release the button and the Instant Pot will automatically start.

14. When the timer goes off after cooking, let the Chile Verde sit in the Instant pot for (at least) an additional 20 minutes until the pressure has reduced and the pot has cooled down a bit. I like to let it sit for about 30 minutes before releasing the rest of the pressure/steam. If you do not manually vent the pot, it will automatically turn to keep warm mode for 10 hours.

15. You may crush the meat up a bit with a potato masher if you like the chunks to be smaller and bits of meat to fall off into the sauce.

16. Serve with guac, chopped avocado, fresh lime, and tortillas.

Philly Cheesesteak Soup:

Put the streets of Philly in your soup pot with this enticing combination of beef, mushrooms, and provolone cheese.

Not many people may know this, but a Philly Cheesesteak is Philadelphia cheesesteak. This famous cheesesteak recipe originated in Philadelphia and has been known all over the United States, and even the rest of the world as it has become the favorite food of many.

So what makes this dish special then? Why is it that many people from around the world favor this taste over the other cheesesteak recipes?

Perhaps one of the distinct characteristics of Philly cheesesteak is its meat. The meat slices in this recipe are generally thinly sliced top round or rib eye. Although other types of meat can be used for this dish, the top round and rib eye are most preferred. The meat slices are ensured to retain its juices as these are cooked at medium temperature on a lightly oiled griddle. As soon as the steak slices turn brown, these are quickly scrambled into finer pieces using a flat spatula. To make sure that these steak slices are perfectly cooked, these are often placed on top of fried onions. Aside from preventing the steak to be overcooked, the onions provide a pleasing aroma and a fusion of tastes into the meat.

While there can be many types of bread used in this dish, Philly cheesesteaks use Vilotti-Pisanelli rolls or Amoroso rolls. Although there are many different variations of the Philly cheesecake as claimed by some locals and sources, the one thing that practically nearly all of these people agree on is the type of bread that would be perfect for a mouthwatering meal. Certainly, almost everyone agrees that regardless of the type of cheese and meat that you prefer for your version of this cheesesteak, it must be all piled up on top of an Amoroso roll. Such that, if you are looking for the original Philly recipe, one item that would confirm its authenticity is the Amoroso roll.

On the other hand, no cheesesteak is ever complete without the cheese. The choice of cheese can vary depending on the preferences of the individual, but the most commonly used cheeses are Mozzarella, Provolone, American cheese, and Cheez Whiz. While the original 1930 version of the recipe does not include Cheez Whiz in the choices of cheese, it has become a common option as soon as it was marketed out commercially in 1952. In fact, according to to most connoisseurs, Cheez Whiz is the secret ingredient in creating delicious cheesesteaks.

Over the years, the recipe has evolved into several variations. One popular variation is the buffalo chicken cheesesteak, which uses buffalo wings sauce and blue cheese dressing. Yet, another famous variation is the hoagie, which contains mayonnaise, tomato, and lettuce.

This recipe may have changed from one version to another, but the Philly cheesesteak will always remain as the best tasting original recipe ever.

Italian Sausage Soup with Tomatoes and Zoodles:

Enjoy a guilt-free bowl of Italian-style zoodles, bursting with oregano awesomeness.

There are several different foods from the Italian culture that are worth noting, but it is the Italian sausage that seems to come to mind so many times. This meat is delightful, and it is a meat that has a place in many great dishes not only back in the motherland but North America too. This meat is available just about anywhere today, and there are various forms of the sausage that you can purchase in most grocery stores let alone the butcher shops. Finding the type of sausage that pleases you is not difficult; you are just going to have to try as many as you can.

Excellent for Sauces

When it comes to Italian pasta sauce, you are going to find some meat that will be added. One such meat that graces a wonderful sauce is the Italian sausage. This meat can be spicy and it is very easy to cut, making it a great meat to work with and an excellent choice. With mild, medium, and hot on the menu you are not going to struggle to find a decent meal for your sauce. These sausages can be cut into small disks or even chunks that are great to stew within a pasta or tomato sauce for hours at a time. Usually, the meat is not cooked prior, as it is going to stew for a great number of hours within the broth. This will not only instill the sauce within the meat, but it will also bring out the great flavors of the meat into the sauce.

Finding the Right Sausage

It is not difficult today to find good Italian sausage, and depending on how much you are looking for and what variety you should have no troubles at all locating it. Most grocery and specialty stores carry this sausage today, and if you are fortunate enough to have an Italian butcher shop near your home, you can find it there. This is not to say that you cannot find it elsewhere; it is simply to imply that there are great chances of finding this sausage at the aforementioned locations first. Most deli's whether they are Italian or not will usually carry this sausage as it was very popular. Many sub shops and sandwich shops will carry it now as well, as they usually have a hot Italian sub on the menu.

Other Uses

Italian sausage is not solely reserved for Italian food today, as you will find many restaurants and sandwich shops all having this meat on their roster of fine foods. The sausage is relatively cheap, and you can bet that there are more than a few people that eat in these locations that consider it a favorite. This meat is easy to prepare, and you have almost endless options when it comes to its uses. Soups and stews are always popular with this meat in them, as too are great casseroles and baked foods.

Low-Carb Smoked Salmon Chowder:

If lox bagels are your vice, you'll weep with joy over this chowder, which has all the same flavors without the carbs.

It can be really hard to diet sometimes, especially when you're trying to cut back on your favorite foods. There are plenty of diet foods out there but so many of them are tasteless and bland that it can seem more like you're torturing yourself then that you're helping yourself when you eat them. Do you ever wish that you could find healthy food that was low in carbs and good for you? Well, look no further than low carb smoked salmon for your next meal!

Low carb smoked salmon is a wonderful food when you're on a diet because it has everything you need to stay healthy and stay on your plan. One of the great advantages of smoked salmon is that it tastes great. It's everything you've been missing since you went on a diet, with none of the guilt! It's great to have the rich, full taste of smoked salmon as part of a snack or a meal, and know that it's good for you! And there are so many different ways to enjoy it!

Smoked salmon has many great health benefits. Of course, it's low in carbohydrates? But what does that mean for you? We all hear the benefits of a low carb diet, but low carb smoked salmon is a really smart way to take advantage of that diet. By cutting down on your carbohydrates, you're taking away a major way that your body produces sugar. That sugar, when there is too much of it, is then stored as fat, and we all know where that ends up!

Smoked salmon is also great for you because it's full of Omega three fatty acids. No, that's not a contradiction. Carbs turn into the bad type of fat, the kind that ends up on your stomach and thighs. But low carb smoked salmon is full of omega-three fatty acids, which doctors say are essential for heart health. So, with smoked salmon, you can get all the heart-healthy benefits you're looking for, without gaining the weight that you're not. Who woulddon't want to snack on something like that, that also tastes great!

When you try low carb smoked salmon, don't be shocked by how good it tastes. You may have started to think that anything that advertises itself as low carb must taste like cardboard, but it's not true. Processes bars designed to be low carb are also often awful, but smoked salmon is naturally low in carbohydrates, which means you get its natural delicious flavors. It's also a high protein snack, which means it can give you the energy boost you need to get to the gym, or just get through your day.

The next time you wonder what you could use to spice up your boring diet food, think about low carb smoked salmon. It's a snack that tastes decadent, but is still good for you, a combination everyone loves. It's a good way to get protein for energy, and treat your heart as well!

MEATLESS & VEGGIE KETO SOUP RECIPES

SAVORY PUMPKIN SOUP

With the right approach, you can have pumpkin on a keto diet — and this keto soup recipe is one tasty example of how to do it. Pureed pumpkin blends with creamy coconut milk and warm spices for a silky, satisfying meal with less than 5 net carbs. Make it more Bulletproof with pastured broth and Ceylon cinnamon, plus skip the nutmeg and garlic (or avoid enjoying often).

Ingredients

- 6 cups sugar pumpkin peeled and cubed

- 6 cups butternut squash peeled and cubed

- 64 oz chicken broth 8 cups

- 1 1/2 tsp ground black pepper

- 1 1/2 tsp dried marjoram

- 1/4 tsp cayenne pepper or more if you like it hot

- 3 cloves of minced garlic

- 1 large chopped yellow onion

- 2 T butter

- 3 cups half and half

- Sea salt to taste

- Dried cranberries and salted roasted pistachios for garnish optional

Instructions

Use a "Y" peeler to peel pumpkin and butternut squash. Cut in half and use a spoon to scrape out seeds. Cut into 1" cubes. In a large pot, bring broth, squash, pumpkin, marjoram, black pepper, and cayenne pepper to boiling. Simmer for 15 minutes or until butternut squash and pumpkin are very tender. While squash is simmering, sauté onion in a small pan with garlic and butter till soft. When squash has cooked for 15 minutes add sautéed onions and a half and a half to squash mixture, stir. Allow cooling until just warm. Ladle into a blender and very carefully puree until smooth. You will have to split into portions to fit your blender. Return to pot and heat thru. Do not bring it to a boil again. Add salt to taste and more cayenne if desired. Garnish and serve.

HEARTY GREEN SOUP

Winter colds are pretty much unavoidable... I'd be lying if I said this soup was some "magic cure" for winter sickness (if anyone finds that... can you let me know?), but I believe filling ourselves with as much good, healthy food as possible can only be a good thing.

This simple soup is packed full of lovely flavor from the potato and carrot base, the fresh thyme and the lentils. You can use whatever your favorite dark leafy greens are, or whatever is in the season for you!

You're sure to feel cozy and warm inside after a bowl of this!

Ingredients

- 1 White Onion
- 2 cloves garlic
- 2 Large Potatoes (approx. 500g)
- 2 Carrots
- 1-liter Vegetable Stock
- 1/2 cup (100g) Green or Brown Lentils
- 1 tbsp Fresh Thyme (chopped)
- 3-4 Large Swiss Chard Leaves (or kale)
- salt and pepper (for seasoning)

Instructions

1. Dice the carrot and potato into small chunks. Finely dice the onion and mince the garlic.

2. Heat a large stockpot on medium heat and add a little oil into the bottom. Once hot, saute the onion until translucent (2-3 minutes) then add the garlic and cook for 1 more minute.

3. After 1 minute, add in the potatoes and carrots and stir to coat with the onion mixture. Add in the thyme too and cook

everything together for 5 minutes until the carrot and potato just begin to soften.

4. Add the vegetable stock and lentils, cover and simmer for 25-30 minutes, until the vegetables and lentils are completely cooked.

5. Take off the heat and if desired, use a stick blender to roughly blend the soup. I like to leave some chunks in for texture, but if you prefer completely smooth soup, you can blend it more.

6. Once blended, chop the swiss chard (or whatever kind of dark leafy green you are using) into strips, and stir into the soup. The heat from the soup will wilt the greens so there's no need to cook them.

Recipe Notes

Soup will keep in an airtight container in the fridge for up to 5 days, or up to 3 months in the freezer.

AIP ASPARAGUS SOUP

The reason I love this soup so much (and ate it for 2 days straight), is that it reminds me of one of my favorite non-AIP soups; Split Pea with Ham. Remember that oldie but goodie? You all may know by now that I love hacking AIP food. If you follow me on Instagram would see that I am constantly trying to make eating AIP easy, easy, easy and making a lot of uber time-saving AIP One-Dish Wonders (everything in one dish, about 15 min. prep time and it all cooks in the oven together). Time is at a premium for me these days! I am ALL about the shortcuts.

But, back to the soup. It has 5 ingredients. And, it is so creamy you would think that there was cream in it. I did use my Blendtec blender which may make a difference in how effectively the asparagus was blended without having random asparagus fibers which I think makes the soup a little on the sad side. I find that being sure you trim the root-ends of the asparagus at least 2-3 inches makes a big difference. If you don't have a pressure cooker or a high-speed blender, don't despair. You can do stovetop and a regular blend for this recipe too! I shared a secret skill with all of you in my Creamy Crockpot Lemon Chicken Kale Soup using olive oil in the blending step to emulsify and thicken the soup along with the onion. I used that technique in this recipe too. It SO easy, but massive on flavor!

Ingredients

1. 1 Bunch Asparagus

2. 1 Medium Onion (heaping cup)

3. 5 Slices of Bacon

4. 3 Cups Bone Broth (you can increase or decrease this depending on how thick you like your soup)

5. 3 Tbls olive oil

6. Salt to Taste

Instructions

1. Trim the bottom 2-3 inches off the asparagus and discard. Remove skin from onion and roughly chop it. Cut bacon into 2-inch sized pieces. Add asparagus, bacon, onion, and stock to the pressure cooker and bring to full pressure for 10 minutes. (If you don't have a pressure cooker, then cook

everything on the stovetop on medium-high heat for 40 minutes)

2. Release pressure and carefully pour it into the blender. Add olive oil. Put on the lid, and then put a dish towel over the blender lid. (be so careful! remember to use a towel on the lid and be sure lid is on tight...also start your blender on the slowest speed!)

3. Blend on high for 2 minutes.

4. Taste for salt.

5. You can serve immediately or cook more on a low simmer.

ANTI-INFLAMMATORY EGG DROP SOUP

This egg drop soup is perfect for chilly autumn days. It cannot be any easier and takes less than 20 minutes to prepare. Just like my Keto Golden Milk, this recipe uses turmeric and ginger. Turmeric is a powerful adaptogen providing a myriad of health benefits: it's immune-boosting and has antioxidant and anti-inflammatory effects.

Ingredients (makes 6 servings)

• 2 quarts (2 l) chicken stock or vegetable stock or bone broth - you can make your own

• 1 tbsp freshly grated turmeric or 1 tsp ground turmeric

• 1 tbsp freshly grated ginger or 1 tsp ground ginger

• 2 cloves garlic, minced

• 1 small chile pepper, sliced (14 g/ 0.5 oz)

• 2 tbsp coconut aminos

- 2 cups sliced brown mushrooms (144 g/ 5.1 oz)

- 4 cups chopped Swiss chard or spinach (144 g/ 5.1 oz)

- 4 large eggs

- 2 medium spring onions, sliced (30 g/ 1.1 oz)

- 2 tbsp freshly chopped cilantro

- 1 tsp salt or to taste (I like pink Himalayan)

- freshly ground black pepper to taste

- 6 tbsp extra virgin olive oil (90 ml/ 3 fl oz)

Instructions

1. Grate the turmeric and ginger root, slice the chile pepper and mince the garlic cloves.

2. Pour the chicken stock (or vegetable stock) in a large pot and heat over medium heat, until it starts to simmer. Slice the mushrooms, ...

3. chard stalks and chard leaves. Place the turmeric, ginger, garlic, chile pepper, mushrooms, chard stalks, and coconut aminos into the pot and simmer for about 5 minutes.

4. Then add the sliced chard leaves and cook for another minute. In a bowl, whisk the eggs and slowly pour them into the simmering soup.

5. Keep stirring until the egg is cooked and take off the heat. Chop the cilantro and slice the spring onions. Add them to the pot. Season with salt and pepper to taste.

6. Pour into a serving bowl and drizzle with extra virgin olive oil (a tablespoon per serving). Eat immediately or let it cool down and store in an airtight container for up to 5 days.

LOW-CARB VEGETARIAN RAMEN

Make a savory meatless meal using this keto soup recipe. Every bite is packed with veggies like zucchini noodles and cabbage, all in a spicy broth seasoned with curry paste and ginger. Every serving is 11 net carbs, so you can make room for veggies without maxing out your macros.

Ramen Ingredients:

• 4 cups of filtered water

• 1 tablespoon sugar-free red curry paste, or chili-infused oil (ingredients below)

• 2 cups full-fat canned coconut milk (BPA-free)

• 1 tablespoon coconut oil (exclude if preparing chili-infused oil)

• 1 cup purple cabbage, chopped

• 1 cup large shredded rainbow carrots

• 1 cup halved Brussel sprouts, halved

• 4 pastured eggs

• 2 large zucchinis, spiralized

• 2 teaspoon ground ginger

• 1 teaspoon ground turmeric

• 1 teaspoon garlic powder

- Himalayan salt and pepper to taste

- Optional: Fresh lime juice or cilantro to garnish

More from Bulletproof

- Easy Blender Pumpkin Collagen Bread

- 20 Low-Carb Fish Recipes You Can Make in a Flash

- Lower-Carb Cauliflower Fried Rice

- Low-Carb Paleo Almond Flour Pie Crust

Chili-infused oil ingredients:

- 1 tablespoon coconut oil

- 1/4 – 1/2 teaspoon red chili flakes

Instructions:

1. In a large pot, add water and bring to a boil.

2. While water begins boiling, prepare chili-infused oil (if using). Heat oil in a small pan on medium heat. When hot, add chili flakes and gently sizzle for about 5 minutes. Remove from heat and set aside.

3. When water is boiling, add coconut milk and spices and reduce heat to medium.

4. Add cabbage, carrots, and brussels sprouts, plus coconut oil and curry paste (if not using chili-infused oil).

5. Cook for about 20 minutes, or until vegetables are tender.

6. While cooking, soft boils the eggs. Fill a separate small pot with water and bring to a boil. Once boiling, reduce to a rapid simmer, add eggs, and cook for 6 minutes. Remove

immediately and drench in ice water to stop the cooking process.

7. When vegetables in the pot are tender, add zucchini and cook for 3-4 more minutes.

8. Serve vegetarian ramen with a peeled and halved soft-boiled egg, lime juice, cilantro, and chili-infused oil.

Note on ingredients: Cabbage and brussels sprouts are high in oxalates—a type of antinutrient that can cause muscle pain, kidney stones, or thyroid imbalances. To reduce oxalates, you can lightly steam these veggies, drain the cooking water, and then add to the pot instead of boiling. All pepper is suspect on the Bulletproof Diet and highly susceptible to performance-robbing mold toxins. To reduce your risk, omit it or find a fresh, high-quality variety.

SPRING SOUP WITH POACHED EGG

Romaine lettuce... in a soup? Try it to believe it: This super-simple keto soup recipe needs just four ingredients, plus you poach your eggs in the soup broth to save time. To make this soup Bulletproof, simply use pastured broth and eggs — every serving is still just 4 net carbs.

Ingredients

• 2 eggs

• 32 oz (1 quart) chicken broth

• 1 head of romaine lettuce, chopped

• salt to taste

Instructions

1. Bring the chicken broth to a boil.

2. Turn down the heat and poach the 2 eggs in the broth for 5 minutes (for a slightly-runny egg).

3. Remove the eggs and place each into a bowl.

4. Add the chopped romaine lettuce into the broth and cook for a few minutes until slightly wilted.

5. Ladle, the broth with the lettuce, into the bowls.

CREAMY LEEK & SALMON SOUP

Skip the heavy meats and try seafood in your soup instead. This keto recipe gets the delicate flavor from leeks and a creamy coconut-based broth, all with bite-size chunks of salmon. Make this soup more Bulletproof with wild-caught salmon and pastured chicken broth, plus skip the garlic.

Ingredients

• 2 tbs avocado oil

• 4 leeks, washed, trimmed and sliced into crescents

• 3 cloves garlic, minced

• 6 cups seafood OR chicken broth

• 2 tsp dried thyme leaves

• 1 lb salmon, in bitesize pieces (thawed frozen salmon works well here)

• 1 3/4 cup coconut milk

- Salt & pepper to taste (omit pepper for AIP)

Instructions

1. Heat the avocado oil in a large saucepan or dutch oven at low-medium heat.

2. Add the chopped leeks and garlic and cook until slightly softened.

3. Pour in the stock and add the thyme. Simmer for about 15 minutes and season to taste with salt and pepper.

4. Add the salmon and the coconut milk to the pan. Bring back up to a gentle simmer and cook until the fish is opaque and tender.

5. Serve immediately!

CREAMY CAULIFLOWER SOUP

This chunky, chowder-like soup gets a creamy flair from a few rich tablespoons of butter, and savory texture from veggies like celery and carrots. Just 12 net carbs per serving. For a more Bulletproof approach to this keto soup recipe, use grass-fed butter, swap the olive oil for avocado oil, skip the onion and garlic, trade cornstarch for arrowroot starch, and trade milk for extra broth.

Ingredients

- 1 head of cauliflower
- 2 tablespoons olive oil
- 1 medium white onion, peeled and diced

- 5 cloves garlic, peeled and minced

- 3 cups Kitchen Basics Organic Vegetable Stock

- 2 sprigs fresh thyme

- 3 cups milk (I used 2%, but any kind of milk will do)

- 1/2 cup freshly grated Parmesan cheese

- Kosher salt and freshly-craked black pepper

- optional garnishes: sauteed cauliflower florets (*see instructions below), roasted chickpeas, fresh thyme leaves, extra Parmesan, and/or extra black pepper

Instructions

1. Begin by prepping your cauliflower. Remove and discard the outer leaves and trim off the stem. Quarter the cauliflower by using a knife to slice it down the middle of the stem, separating it into four sections. Separate the core from the florets. Roughly chop the florets, and then thinly slice the core. Set aside. (Also, if you'd like to garnish the soup with a bit of sautéed cauliflower, set aside 1 cup of florets for later use. See instructions below.)

2. Heat oil in a large stockpot over medium-high heat. Add the onion and sauté for 5 minutes, until soft and translucent, stirring occasionally. Stir in the garlic and continue to sauté for 1-2 more minutes, until fragrant.

3. Add in the chopped cauliflower, vegetable stock, and thyme, and stir to combine. Continue cooking until the mixture reaches a simmer. Then reduce heat to medium-low, cover, and continue simmering for about 20-25 minutes, or until the cauliflower is tender. Remove the thyme sprigs.

4. Using either an immersion blender or transferring the soup in batches to a traditional blender (be careful not to fill it very full when working with hot soups), puree the soup until smooth.

5. Stir in the milk and Parmesan, and season the soup to taste with salt and black pepper.

6. Serve immediately, topped with your desired garnishes if desired.

Notes

If you would like to garnish the soup with sauteed cauliflower, heat 1 tablespoon of butter (or oil) in a medium saute pan over medium-high heat. Add the cauliflower florets and sauté for 3-4 minutes, or until they are tender and slightly golden on the outside.

NO-COOK REFRESHING MINT AVOCADO CHILLED SOUP

This bright and creamy soup recipe takes just minutes to prepare and uses filling ingredients like avocado, romaine lettuce, coconut milk, lime juice, and fresh mint. Stay Bulletproof and simply use full-fat canned coconut milk from a BPA-free can.

No-Cook Refreshing Mint Avocado Chilled Soup Recipe — Step-by-step Instructions

Step 1:

Cut a ripe avocado in half. Remove the stone, and scoop out the avocado flesh. Place into a blender. (This dish can be made in pretty much any blender, but you might have a bit more trouble getting it to blend well with a cheap magic bullet type blender).

Step 2:

Squeeze the lime juice into the blender – 1 tablespoon of lime juice (approximately the juice from half a lime). Add the lime juice quickly to prevent the avocado from turning brown (oxidizing).

Step 3:

Add in the romaine lettuce leaves and mint leaves to the blender as well. Then pour in the chilled coconut milk and a bit of salt (you can add more salt in later if you wish). If you use coconut milk from the cans, then shake it well before use and dilute it with some water. If you use the coconut milk from the cartons, then make sure you use one without added sugar.

Step 4:

Blend well. Taste it and add in more lime juice or salt if you prefer. Chill the soup for a few minutes and then serve.

Ingredients

1. 1 medium ripe avocado

2. 2 romaine lettuce leaves

3. 1 cup (240 ml) coconut milk, chilled (from cartons or else dilute the canned coconut milk)

4. 1 Tablespoon (15 ml) lime juice

5. 20 fresh mint leaves

6. Salt to taste

SUPERFOOD KETO SOUP

Use this keto recipe for an easy way to balance your micronutrients. It uses veggies like cauliflower, watercress, and fresh spinach to create a creamy, bright green concoction. To stay Bulletproof, skip the onions and garlic (or replace with fresh herbs), and steam cauliflower and spinach separately before adding to the recipe.

INGREDIENTS:

• 1 medium head cauliflower (400 g / 14.1 oz)

• 1 medium white onion (110 g / 3.9 oz)

• 2 cloves garlic

• 1 bay leaf, crumbled

• 150 g watercress (5.3 oz)

• 200 g fresh spinach (7.1 oz) or frozen spinach (220 g / 7.8 oz)

• 1-liter vegetable stock or bone broth or chicken stock – you can make your own (4 cups / 1 quart)

• 1 cup cream or coconut milk (240 ml / 8 fl oz) + 6 tbsp for garnish

• 1/4 cup ghee or coconut oil – you can make your ghee (55 g / 1.9 oz)

• 1 tsp salt or to taste (I like pink Himalayan rock salt)

• freshly ground black pepper

INSTRUCTIONS:

1. Peel and finely dice the onion and garlic. Place in a soup pot or a Dutch oven greased with ghee and cook over medium-high heat until slightly browned. Wash the spinach and watercress and set aside.

2. Cut the cauliflower into small florets and place them in the pot with browned onion. Add crumbled bay leaf. Cook for about 5 minutes and mix frequently.

3. Add the spinach and watercress and cook until wilted for just about 2-3 minutes.

4. Pour in the vegetable stock and bring to a boil. Cook until the cauliflower is crisp-tender and pours in the cream (or coconut milk).

5. Season with salt and pepper. Take off the heat and using a hand blender, pulse until smooth and creamy.

SPICY KETO SOUP RECIPES

LOW-CARB THAI CURRIED BUTTERNUT SQUASH SOUP

This zippy keto soup recipe uses red curry paste for a spicy kick, then balances the heat with creamy coconut milk and pureed butternut squash. Each serving is 8 net carbs and packed with flavor. To make this soup more Bulletproof, simply skip the onions and garlic.

Ingredients

- 1 tablespoon coconut oil

- 1 small onion peeled and chopped

- 2 cloves garlic crushed

- 2 tablespoons red curry paste

- 1/4 teaspoon cayenne pepper (more or less to taste)

- 3 cups low-salt chicken bone broth

- 1 can coconut milk

• 12 ounces butternut squash peeled, seeds removed, and cut into large chunks

• sea salt to taste

• 1/4 cup cilantro chopped

• additional cilantro or coconut flakes for garnish (optional)

Instructions

1. Preheat a dutch oven or a soup pot over medium heat. Add coconut oil. When the coconut oil has melted, add onions. Cook onions, stirring frequently, until they appear translucent and the edges begin to brown.

2. Stir in the garlic, red curry pastes, and cayenne pepper. Cook until fragrant, about one minute.

3. Stir in the broth, coconut milk, and butternut squash. Bring mixture to a simmer. Simmer, uncovered, until the squash is very tender.

4. Puree soup in batches using a blender, or puree in the pot using an immersion blender.

5. Stir in cilantro. Taste and add sea salt to taste. If desired, garnish with additional cilantro or coconut flakes.

KETO INSTANT POT CHICKEN ENCHILADA SOUP

With the quick-cooking power of the Instant Pot, you can have this zesty soup ready in about 30 minutes. For 9 net carbs, every bowlful contains satisfying chunks of chicken, peppers, and onions in a spicy tomato broth. If you're sensitive to nightshades, skip this recipe to stay Bulletproof — otherwise, omit garlic and onions, use pastured chicken and broth, and use apple cider vinegar instead of white wine vinegar.

How to Make Keto Chicken Enchilada Soup?

This one is so easy; it almost feels like you're cheating. But for a keto version, we need to skip all the beans and corn and grain-based thickeners and focus mostly on the chicken and the broth.

Boneless skinless chicken is perfect for the instant pot or slow cooker because it cooks easily right in the broth and you don't have to brown it first. Just put it right at the bottom of your pot and once cooking is complete, you should be able to shred it easily.

I used pureed tomatoes from my garden, which I'd stored in the freezer in glass jars. But you can use tomato puree from a can or even diced tomatoes if that's all you can find. Fire-roasted tomatoes would be delicious!

If you're using store-bought taco seasoning for this recipe, make sure to check your labels. Some contain sugars or starches as fillers. I make my own or I buy the bag from Natural Grocers. You could also try Primal Palate, a paleo spice mix.

Since some of my favorite enchiladas are ones with a sour cream sauce, I opted for sour cream to make the broth rich and creamy. Adding sour cream straight to a hot liquid can cause it to curdle a bit so I recommend removing about a cup of the hot broth and whisking it into the sour cream, then whisking the whole thing back into the pot.

This is such a simple and straightforward soup with a huge flavor impact. And it's wonderful to be able to dump all of the ingredients in without too many extra steps.

Ingredients

- 2 lbs boneless skinless chicken thighs or breasts

- 2 cups pureed tomatoes (canned is fine)

- 1/2 cup chopped onion

- 2 jalapeños, diced

- 1/4 cup butter

- 3 tbsp taco seasoning

- 3/4 tsp salt

- 5 cups chicken broth

- 3/4 cup sour cream

Instructions

1. Place the chicken, tomatoes, onion, jalapeños, butter, taco seasoning and salt in the bottom of an Instant Pot or slow cooker. Pour the broth over the top.

2. For, the Instant Pot, seal the lid and make sure the vent is on the seal. Set to the Soup Function for 20 minutes. Let the pressure release naturally for 15 minutes.

3. For a slow cooker, place the lid on and set too low for 6 to 8 hours or high for 3 to 4 hours.

4. When cooking is complete, remove the chicken to a plate. Remove about 1 cup of the hot broth to a bowl and whisk in the sour cream, then whisk this combo back into the pot.

5. Shred the chicken with two forks and add back into the pot. Adjust seasonings to taste. Serve hot with cheese and chopped avocados.

KETO LOW-CARB CHILI

This meaty chili has just the right amount of heat, thanks to ingredients like chili powder, green chiles, and cumin. Stay a little more Bulletproof with this recipe and use grass-fed ground beef, swap Worcestershire with coconut aminos, and skip the onions and garlic. If you're sensitive to nightshades like peppers and onions, try a different keto soup recipe.

Ingredients

- 2 lbs 80/20 ground beef
- 4 garlic cloves minced
- 1/2 small onion diced
- 10 oz can Rotel Tomatoes
- 28 oz can crushed tomatoes
- 1 1/4 tablespoon cumin
- 2 1/2 tablespoon chili powder
- 1 tablespoon curry powder
- 28 oz beef broth
- 1 1/2 teaspoon salt
- 2 tsp pepper
- 1 tablespoon red pepper flakes optional
- 1 tablespoon hot sauce optional

Instructions

1. Brown ground beef, onions, and minced garlic together in a large saucepan.

2. Drain (if desired) then return to saucepan.

3. Add all other ingredients to the ground beef mixture and bring to a boil.

4. Reduce to low and simmer uncovered for 1 1/2 to 2 hours or until chili reaches desired thickness.

5. Top each bowl with sour cream, grated cheese, jalapenos if desired.

INSTANT POT OR SLOW COOKER SPICY BEEF AND BROCCOLI ZOODLE SOUP

With a simple ginger beef broth, tender steak tips and zoodles serve the perfect starring roles in this low-carb soup recipe. For, a more Bulletproof adaptation, skip the mushrooms, use pastured beef and broth, choose coconut aminos, and use a hot sauce made with apple cider vinegar.

Ingredients

• 2 tbsp avocado oil

• 3 tbsp fresh ginger minced

• 2 cloves garlic minced

• 1.5 lbs top sirloin steak tips about 1-inch pieces

• 2 heaping cups of fresh broccoli florets

• 8 oz sliced Bella mushrooms

• 6 cups beef broth

- 1/4 cup apple cider vinegar

- 1/4 cup coconut aminos or soy sauce

- 1/4 cup buffalo hot sauce or sriracha*

- 1 large zucchini spiralized for noodles

- 1/3 cup chopped fresh green onion

Instructions

For the Instant Pot:

1. Select the saute function on your Instant Pot. Once hot, add avocado oil, ginger, garlic, and steak tips. Cook for a few minutes, until the beef, is lightly browned on each side, and garlic/ginger is flavorful. Select cancel.

2. Now add broccoli, mushrooms, beef broth, vinegar, coconut aminos or soy sauce, and hot sauce. You can also save the broccoli and add with zoodles after the soup has cooked if you want the broccoli to be crisper. Stir and secure the lid.

3. Select the manual function on your Instant Pot. Cook on high pressure for 8 minutes. Then use a quick release to let the steam out.

4. Now open the lid, adjust to the more hot sauce for a spicier variation. Add in the spiralized zucchini, top with fresh green onion, and serve hot.

For the Slow Cooker:

1. Heat a large skillet to medium heat. Once hot, add oil and cook the ginger and garlic for about 2 minutes. Add beef to

the pan, and cook for about 5 minutes until each side is lightly browned (it does not need to be cooked all the way).

2. Toss beef, ginger, and garlic inside your slow cooker. Add broccoli, mushrooms, broth, vinegar, soy sauce or coconut aminos, and hot sauce. Broccoli can also be saved until toward the end of cooking time for a crisper taste. Set your slow cooker to low, and cook for 4-5 hours or until beef is tender and soup is flavorful. Add in additional hot sauce for a spicier variation.

3. Add in spiralized zucchini, and serve with fresh green onion.

Recipe Notes

*Use either buffalo sauce or sriracha. If following a Paleo or Whole30 diet, Sriracha is not approved and buffalo sauce should be used in its place.

KETO INSTANT POT THAI SHRIMP SOUP

Red curry paste, lemongrass, ginger, and coconut milk create a fragrant broth for this keto soup recipe, all topped with tender shrimp. This soup contains only 4 net carbs per serving and cooks up in under 20 minutes using the Instant Pot. Stay Bulletproof and use wild-caught shrimp and grass-fed butter, omit the mushrooms, and only enjoy garlic and onion once in a while.

Ingredients:

• 2 tbsp unsalted butter or ghee, divided in half

• ½lb (225g) medium uncooked shrimp, peeled and deveined

• ½ yellow onion, diced

- 2 cloves garlic, minced

- 4 cups chicken broth

- 2 tbsp fresh lime juice

- 2 tbsp fish sauce, this brand is whole30 compliant

- 2½ tsp red curry paste, like this one

- 1 tbsp coconut aminos (paleo whole30) or can use 1 tbsp tamari sauce for low carb

- 1 stalk lemongrass, bruised (smashed) and finely chopped

- 1 cup sliced fresh white mushrooms

- 1 tbsp grated fresh ginger root

- 1 tsp sea salt

- ½ tsp freshly ground black pepper

- 1 (13.66-ounce) can unsweetened, full-fat coconut milk (this brand is whole30 compliant)

- 3 tbsp chopped fresh cilantro

Directions:

1. Press the Sauté button once. Once the inner pot becomes hot, add 1 tbsp butter. Once butter is melted, add the shrimp and stir until shrimp turns pink and begins to curl. Immediately transfer shrimp to a medium bowl. Set aside.

2. Add the remaining 1 tbsp butter to the inner pot. Once butter is melted, add onions and garlic and sauté until garlic is fragrant and onions become translucent. Press Cancel to turn off the heat.

3. Add chicken broth, lime juice, fish sauce, red curry paste, coconut aminos or tamari sauce, lemongrass, mushrooms, grated ginger root, sea salt, and black pepper. Stir to combine.

4. Cover, lock the lid and flip the steam release handle to the Sealing position. Select Pressure Cook on High, and set the cooking time for 5 minutes. When the cooking time is complete, allow the pressure to release naturally for 5 minutes (Don't touch the pot for 5 minutes), and then carefully quick release the remaining pressure by flipping the steam release handle to "Venting." Press Cancel to turn off the heat.

5. Remove the lid. Add shrimp and coconut milk to the pot, and stir.

6. Press the Sauté button twice ("more or high" setting will light up), and let the soup come to a boil. Once boiling Press Cancel to turn off the heat. Let the soup rest for 2 minutes in the pot.

7. Ladle the soup into bowls, sprinkle cilantro over the top to garnish and serve.

Chapter Three
Easy-to-do recipes

One of my oldest friends recently admitted that she has trouble in the kitchen. She asked me if I had any simple recipes that she could make for her family. I thought that I would help her out by assembling a list of easy recipes for beginners – a collection of foolproof recipes that anyone can successfully make.

Sweet and Spicy Sausage Farfalle

Sweet and Spicy Sausage and Farfalle is a 20-minute dinner recipe that I grew up eating and fell in love with again as a adult. It is one of the easiest recipes you can ask for, and the speedy preparation time makes it a perfect weeknight dinner option.

How to Make Sweet and Spicy Sausage and Farfalle – a 20-minute dinner recipe:

Sweet and Spicy Sausage and Farfalle

Sweet and Spicy Sausage and Farfalle is a recipe that I grew up eating and fell in love with again as an adult. It is one of the easiest recipes you can ask for, and the speedy preparation time makes it a perfect weeknight dinner option. When I was growing up, I couldn't understand why we had sweet and spicy sausage and farfalle for dinner all the time. As an adult, I get it! This is the little recipe that can feed your family of 4-5 with just 20 minutes to total preparation time. Plus, the ingredients are all super cheap. It makes perfect sense that my Mom made this recipe to feed our family of five frequently.

Ingredients

- 2 Sweet Italian Sausages 1/2 lb total

- 1/4 cup chopped White Onion

- 2 cloves Garlic

- 1 14.5 oz can have Crushed Tomatoes

- 1/2 cup Heavy Cream

- 1 teaspoon Red Pepper Flakes

- 2 cups Farfalle

- 2 cups Baby Spinach

- 2 tablespoons Parmesan

- 1 tablespoon Olive Oil

Instructions

1. Finely chop the onion and garlic. Slice the ends of the sausage, and push the meat out of the casing, and loosely crumble it up.

2. Bring a pot of salted water to a boil. Once the water has come to a boil, add the pasta. Cook for 7-8 minutes, until al dente. Then drain the pasta and set aside.

3. As soon as you put the water on the boil, start to prepare the rest of this dish. Heat the olive oil in a skillet over medium-high heat. Add the onions and sauté. After 2 minutes, add the sausage and red pepper flakes. For a mild spice add 1/2 teaspoon of red pepper flakes, or add more for extra spice.

4. Brown the sausage, while using a wooden spoon to break it into small pieces.

5. Once the sausage has browned, add the garlic, crushed tomatoes, and cream. Stir together. Let simmer for 2-3 minutes.

6. Add the drained pasta to the sauce, along with the spinach (I tear it up as I add it in). Let the pasta and spinach simmer in the sauce for 2 minutes over medium heat. Serve with a sprinkle of Parmesan.

Recipe Notes

One of the things that I love about this recipe is that you can opt to make it spicy. There are two ways to go about this. First, you can simply use Spicy Italian Sausage instead of Sweet Italian Sausage, or you can add crushed red pepper flakes. If you love spice – you can do both! If you want to eliminate the spicy, just omit the red pepper flakes. I like to add a couple of handfuls of spinach to the sauce right when I mix in the pasta. It helps to turn the pasta into a complete meal. If you wanted, you could add some additional vegetables. Mushrooms and bell peppers would both be excellent additions. I used pork sausage, but you can choose your chicken sausage instead. You could even experiment with using tofu sausage, which I just discovered is a thing! This pasta does reheat well, and I often make a big batch. A single batch is a plenty for four servings, but if you have a larger family – or just really love leftovers – you could make a double batch without adding any additional preparation time.

Easy Beef Pasta Skillet

This rich creamy beef pasta skillet is made with roasted tomatoes, ground beef, and mascarpone cheese to make an irresistible pasta dish. This recipe is centered around fresh summer ingredients, and it can be made in under an hour with just about 30 minutes of active preparation time. I love how this pasta recipe incorporates a good amount of meat and vegetables making it a complete meal.

Ingredients

- 3 cups of Tomatoes (I used Baby Roma)
- 3 tablespoons Olive Oil
- 3 cloves of Garlic, minced
- 8 ounces Sliced Mushrooms
- 3/4 lb Ground Beef (I like Ground Sirloin)
- 1/2 cup Chopped Onion
- 2 tablespoons Tomato Paste
- 1/2 cup Mascarpone
- 8 ounces of Fresh Pasta (I used Rana Tagliatelle)
- 1 tablespoon Fresh Chopped Basil
- 1 tablespoon grated Parmesan

Instructions

1. Start by roasting the tomatoes for 30 minutes. First, heat your oven to 350 degrees. I chopped 1 cup of the tomatoes into quarters, and I left the others right on the vine since I was going to put them in the blender anyway. I always like to line the baking sheet with parchment, it helps the tomatoes to roast more evenly. Then drizzle a tablespoon of olive oil over the tomatoes and generously dust them with salt and pepper.

2. Use the next 30 minutes to catch up on a tv show. You don't need any prep work in the kitchen right now.

3. Once the tomatoes have roasted for 30 minutes, use a slotted spoon to remove the quartered tomatoes and place them in a bowl. Remove the stems from the tomatoes (if you left them on) and pour the whole tomatoes and all of the juices into your blender and liquify. Set aside.

4. Pour 1 tablespoon of olive oil into a skillet over medium heat. Once hot, add the garlic and cook until fragrant. Add the mushrooms. Season with some salt and pepper, and cook for 6-7 minutes, until slightly browned. Then set aside - you can put them in the bowl with the sliced tomatoes if you want.

5. Using the same skillet, add the last tablespoon of olive oil, and then the beef. Season with salt and pepper and use a wooden spoon to stir and break the beef up into small pieces.

6. Once the beef has browned, add the onions to the beef, and cook until they become translucent. Then stir in the liquified tomatoes and the tomato paste. Let simmer and reduce for 2 minutes, then add the mascarpone. As soon as the mascarpone has melted, add the fresh pasta and then the mushrooms and quartered tomatoes.

7. Carefully stir to cover the pasta in the sauce. Let the pasta simmer in the sauce for about 5 minutes until the pasta is al dente. Serve right away. Garnish with the basil and Parmesan.

Creamy Cheddar Mac and Cheese

Everyone loves macaroni and cheese and this recipe for stovetop make and cheese with a crispy panko topping is super simple and can be made in just 20 minutes.

Ingredients

- 2 1/2 cups Medium Shells
- 2 1/2 tablespoons butter
- 2 tablespoons Plain Panko Breadcrumbs
- 2 tablespoons Flour
- 1 1/4 cup 2% Milk
- 1 1/4 cubed Sharp Cheddar
- about 1/2 teaspoon salt
- about 1/4 teaspoon Black Pepper
- a dash of Dry Mustard
- a dash of Paprika

Instructions

1. Bring a pot of salted water to a boil. Once boiling, add the pasta, cooking until al dente according to the directions on the box.

2. Then get to work toasting the breadcrumbs. Melt 1 tablespoon of butter in a small skillet over medium heat. Stir in the breadcrumbs, and continue to stir until the bread crumbs have reached a golden-brown color. Then remove from the heat and set aside.

3. Prepare the sauce next. Melt the remaining butter in a saucepan over medium heat. Once melted, whisk in the flour. Continue whisking until the butter and flour mixture (the roux) is slightly golden.

4. Whisk the milk into the roux. Whisk frequently until the milk comes to a slow and steady boil. Let the mixture boil and thicken for one minute while whisking constantly.

5. Add the cheese to the milk and whiskey until it melts.

6. Season the sauce with the salt and pepper, and a dash of dry mustard and paprika.

7. Drain the pasta and add it to the sauce. Serve with the crispy panko breadcrumbs on top.

Roasted Garlic, Goat Cheese, and Tomato Pasta

A delicious vegetarian pasta recipe that comes together in 40 minutes. I am convinced that roasted garlic makes everything better. Roasted garlic is one of those things that's easy to make a lot of. I always make a whole head of roasted garlic at a time, and then add it to various recipes a few cloves at a time. Recently, I whipped up a quick Roasted Garlic, Goat Cheese, and Tomato Pasta. When I make pasta dishes, I like to use a few simple fresh ingredients. I don't want to over complicate things, so I focused on finding the best ways to use roasted garlic, fresh cherry tomatoes, fresh basil, and goat cheese. The result was a creamy pasta dish bursting with flavor that took just over 30 minutes to prepare.

Ingredients

• 1 head of Garlic

- 2 tablespoons Olive Oil

- 2 cups Cherry Tomatoes (I used red and yellow)

- 1/4 cup Fresh Basil Leaves

- Salt and Pepper

- 12 ounces of Fresh Pasta

- 1 tablespoon butter

- 2 ounces Goat Cheese

- 1/4 cup Pasta Water

Instructions

1. The first thing you need to do is put the garlic in the oven to roast. Slice, the top of the garlic off, exposing the tops of the cloves of garlic. Then place the garlic on two layers of foil - sliced side facing down. Fold the foil up around the garlic. Then drizzle one tablespoon of olive oil over and seal up the foil around the garlic. Place in the oven at 350 degrees.

2. Next prepare the tomatoes. Simply slice the cherry tomatoes in half and place them on a baking sheet. Drizzle the remaining oil over and generously sprinkle with salt and pepper. Roughly chop the basil and sprinkle it over before placing the tomatoes in the oven beside the garlic.

3. Now, you have about 20 minutes to hang out. I read Cooking Light.

4. Ok, hangout time is over. Bring a pot of salted water to a boil.

5. While you are waiting for the water to boil, start working on the roasted garlic goat cheese sauce. Remove the garlic from the oven and carefully unwrap it. Let it cool for a minute before extracting 4-

5 cloves of garlic (or more if you love garlic). The garlic should be very soft; use a fork to mash it.

6. Melt the butter in a skillet over medium heat. Reduce to medium-low heat, and let the butter slowly brown; this brings out more flavor. Once, the butter has started to brown, add the garlic stirring it into the butter. Then add the goat cheese letting it melt. At this point, the mixture will be a thick paste. Remove the tomatoes from the oven, and scoop any tomato liquid at the bottom of the pan into the skillet, thinning out the sauce. Taste the sauce and season with salt and pepper. Then stir the tomatoes into the sauce. Keep warm on low.

7. By now the water should be boiling. Add the pasta to the water and cook according to the directions. Before draining the pasta, remove 1/4 cup of water from the pot.

8. Drain the pasta, and stir the pasta water in the sauce. Add the pasta to the sauce, let simmer for 1 minute, and serve immediately.

Mustard and Mushroom Chicken

A super flavorful chicken recipe that takes just 25 minutes of active preparation time, I have been eating this since I was a kid.

Ingredients

• 2 tablespoons Butter

• 2 cloves Garlic, minced

• 3 tablespoons Flour

• 1 cup Chicken Stock

• 1/2 cup Milk

- 3-4 tablespoons Mustard

- 1 tablespoon Tarragon

- 2 tablespoons Olive Oil

- 8 ounces sliced Mushrooms

- 3 tablespoons White Wine

- 1 Yellow Onion, chopped

- 2 pounds Chicken Breasts

- Flour to dredge the chicken

- Salt and Pepper

Instructions

1. Preheat your oven to 300 degrees. Prepare the chicken by cutting each chicken breast in half and then pounding it with a meat mallet until it has a thin and even thickness.

2. Then start preparing the sauce. Start by melting the butter in a medium saucepan. Stir in the garlic, and let it cook for one minute and then stir in the flour. Stir for another minute. Then slowly add the chicken stock and milk whisk until the butter/flour mixture is completely incorporated. Then bring to a slow boil. Let boil for 1 minute, stirring frequently. This lets the sauce thicken. Then add in the mustard and tarragon. Go ahead and add extra mustard if you like mustard. Set the sauce aside.

3. Heat 1 tablespoon of olive oil in a skillet over medium heat. Add the mushrooms and toss in the olive oil. Sprinkle with salt and pepper. Saute the mushrooms for 4 minutes, and then add the white wine and the onions. Let saute for

another 4 minutes. Then add the mushrooms and onions to the sauce.

4. In a bowl combine about 1/2 cup flour and 1/2 teaspoon of both salt and pepper. Using the same skillet, heat another tablespoon of olive oil over medium-high heat. Once the skillet is hot, dredge the chicken in the flour and place in the skillet. It will only take a couple of minutes to brown on each side. Place the browned chicken in a casserole dish. Continue to brown the chicken in batches, adding more olive oil to the pan as necessary.

5. Once all of the chicken has browned, pour the sauce over, and place it in the oven to bake for 45 minutes.

20 Minute Sesame Chicken

You just need one skillet and 20 minutes to make this delicious sesame chicken. You can easily customize this meal to include all of your favorite veggies too!

Ingredients

• 1.5 pounds Boneless Skinless Chicken Breast

• 3 tablespoons All-Purpose Flour

• 3 teaspoons Sesame Oil

• 3/4 cup Low Sodium Soy Sauce

• 3 cloves of garlic pressed or minced

• 1 teaspoon Peeled Fresh Ginger grated

• 1/2 teaspoon - 1 teaspoon Sriracha to taste

- 2 teaspoons Corn Starch

- 2 cups Sliced Mushrooms

- 1 cup Snow Peas

- 1/2 cup Shredded Carrot I get it from the grocery store salad bar

- 2 teaspoons Sesame Seeds

Instructions

1. Serve with your favorite rice (I used Uncle Ben's Brown and Wild Rice Mix)

2. First, use a knife or kitchen shears to cut the chicken up into pieces that are about 2 bites big.

3. Then toss the chicken in the flour, until it is evenly coated in flour. Next heat a teaspoon of sesame oil in a wok or skillet over medium heat. Once hot, add 1/3 of the chicken and cook each side for 2 minutes until browned. Then cook the rest of the chicken in two more batches, adding another teaspoon of sesame oil to the pan each time. Set the cooked chicken aside in a bowl.

4. Whisk the soy sauce, garlic, ginger, sriracha, and corn starch together and then pour it into the same wok or skillet over medium heat. Add the mushrooms, and let cook for 3 minutes, stirring frequently.

5. Add the chicken, and stir to coat it in the sauce. Cook for another 4 minutes. Lastly, add the snow peas, carrot, and sesame seeds. Cook for 2 minutes. (I used this time to make my Uncle Ben's microwaveable rice).

Sherry Mushroom Chicken

If you want a quick and easy recipe that seems fancy this is your best bet. Chicken breasts are cooked in butter and sherry and then served with a creamy mushroom and sherry sauce. This is always a hit.

Ingredients

- 4 skinless, boneless chicken breast halves

- salt and ground black pepper to taste

- garlic powder, or to taste

- 2 tablespoons butter

- 1 small onion, chopped

- 1 (8 ounces) package sliced fresh mushrooms

- 1 tablespoon olive oil (optional)

- ¼ cup cream sherry

- ¼ cup chicken broth, or as needed (optional)

- 4 slices provolone cheese

Directions

Step 1

Season chicken with salt, pepper, and garlic powder.

Step 2

Heat butter in a skillet over medium heat; cook chicken in the melted butter until no longer pink in the center and juices run clear, 3 to 4 minutes per side. Remove chicken from skillet.

Step 3

Cook and stir onion and mushrooms in the same skillet; add olive oil. Cook until onion and mushrooms are slightly tender, 5 to 10 minutes. Pour sherry and chicken broth into the skillet, and bring to a boil while scraping the browned bits of food off of the bottom of the pan with a wooden spoon, about 2 minutes.

Step 4

Return chicken to the skillet, cover, and simmer chicken and onion mixture until liquid is slightly reduced about 15 minutes. Spoon onion and mushrooms atop each chicken breast and top each with a slice of provolone cheese. Remove skillet from heat; cover skillet until cheese melts, about 5 minutes.

Easy Recipes for Beginners Made with a Slow Cooker:

When someone tells me that they can't cook, I always have the same response, I ask: Do you have a slow cooker? I think everyone needs a slow cooker – they are the best tool for making a lot of food with minimal effort. Here is a few of my favorite crockpot recipes:

4 Ingredient Taco Chicken –

Let's start with the easiest recipe! Throw 4 simple ingredients in a crockpot and a few hours later you have chicken perfect for making tacos! And let's face it – taco night was the best of the week when you were a kid.

Ingredients

• 3 pounds of Boneless Chicken (I used half breast and half thigh)

• 2 cans of Diced Tomatoes with Green Chilis

- 1 packet of Taco Seasoning

- about 1 cup of Chicken Broth

Instructions

1. Pour the diced tomatoes into the slow cooker. Add the taco seasoning and mix thoroughly.

2. Place the chicken in the slow cooker.

3. Pour chicken broth over the chicken until the chicken is submerged in the broth and tomato mixture. Stir to combine everything.

4. Put the lid on the slow cooker and set to low. After 4-5 hours the chicken will fall apart tender.

5. Use a fork to remove the chicken from the slow cooker. Shred with two forks.

6. Use a slotted spoon to scoop the tomatoes out of the sauce, and add to the chicken. Add about 1 cup of the liquid from the slow cooker to the chicken and stir. I discarded the extra liquid in the slow cooker and returned the chicken to the slow cooker and set to the keep warm setting during the party.

Beef Stroganoff

This meal of tender chunks of beef, mushrooms, and onions in a creamy sauce takes just 20 minutes of active preparation time. You just need to quickly brown the beef and saute the mushrooms and onions before throwing everything into a crockpot to cook for 5 hours.

Ingredients

- 600 g / 1.2 lb scotch fillet steak (boneless ribeye) (Note 1)

- 2 tbsp vegetable oil, divided

- 1 large onion (or 2 small onions), sliced

- 300 g / 10 oz mushrooms, sliced (not too thin)

- 40 g / 3 tbsp butter

- 2 tbsp flour (Note 2)

- 2 cups / 500 ml beef broth, preferably salt reduced

- 1 tbsp Dijon mustard

- 150 ml / 2/3 cup sour cream

- Salt and pepper

Serving:

- 250 - 300 g / 8 - 10 oz pasta or egg noodles of choice (Note 3)

• Chopped chives, for garnish (optional)

Instructions

   1.

1. Use your fist (or rolling pin or mallet) to flatten the steaks to about 3/4cm / 1/3" thick. Slice into 5mm / 1/5" strips (cut long ones in half), discarding excess fat.

2. Sprinkle with a pinch of salt and pepper.

3. Heat 1 tbsp oil in a large skillet over high heat. Scatter half the beef in the skillet QUICKLY spread it with tongs. Leave untouched for 30 seconds until browned. Turn beef quickly (as best you can!). Leave untouched for 30 seconds to brown. Immediately remove onto a plate. Don't worry about pink bits and that it will be raw inside.

4. Add remaining 1 tbsp oil and repeat with remaining beef.

5. Turn heat down to medium-high. Add butter, melt. Then add onions, cook for 1 minute, then add mushrooms.

6. Cook mushrooms until golden. Scrape bottom of fry pan to get all the golden bits off (this is flavor!).

7. Add flour, cook, stirring, for 1 minute.

8. Add half the broth while stirring. Once incorporated, add the remaining broth.

9. Stir, then add sour cream and mustard. Stir until incorporated (don't worry if it looks split, sour cream will "melt" as it heats).

10. Bring to simmer, then reduce heat to medium-low. Once it thickens to the consistency of pouring cream (3 - 5 minutes), adjust salt and pepper to taste.

11. Add beef back in (including plate juices). Simmer for 1 minute, then remove from the stove immediately. (Note 4)

12. Serve over pasta, or egg noodles sprinkled with chives if desired.

Recipe Notes:

1. The best cut of beef for a stroganoff - use decent to good quality quick-cooking cut of beef such as:

boneless rib eye (aka scotch fillet)

boneless sirloin, sirloin steak tips

beef tenderloin

I don't recommend beef round steak (aka topside), skirt, flat iron, hanger.

Pork can also be used - pork stroganoff is found in Russia too.

2. Flour - any is fine here; I use plain white flour (all-purpose). Or use 1 tbsp cornstarch/cornflour (for Gluten-free stroganoff sauce)

3. Serving - I like serving this with short pasta, rather than long pasta. Easier to eat. It's also great with mashed potato, rice, polenta - anything that's suitable to slop up all that gravy!

4. Sauce thickness: You can make sauce thinner with a touch of water if you want, but DO NOT keep simmering to thicken once the beef is added, it will overcook the beef.

5. Storage - 3 to 4 days in the fridge, also freezes fine. Thaw fully then reheat carefully, being sure not to overcook the beef!

6. Nutrition per serving, assuming 5 servings (serves 4 hearty servings or 5 sensible servings), excludes pasta.

BBQ Pulled Pork Sandwiches

I love this recipe because you can customize your sandwiches with your favorite toppings. Just like the other crockpot recipes, you just need to throw a bunch of ingredients together and let your meal cook.

Ingredients

- 1 boneless pork loin roast (2 pounds)
- 1 cup barbecue sauce
- 1/4 cup chopped onion
- 2 garlic cloves, minced
- 1/2 teaspoon ground cumin
- 1/8 teaspoon pepper
- 16 slices sourdough bread
- 1 chipotle pepper in adobo sauce, chopped

- 3/4 cup mayonnaise

- 8 slices cheddar cheese

- 2 plum tomatoes, thinly sliced

Directions

1. Place pork in a 3-qt. slow cooker. Combine the barbecue sauce, onion, garlic, cumin, salt, and pepper; pour over pork. Cover and cook on low for 6-7 hours or until meat is tender. Remove meat. Shred with two forks and return to slow cooker; heat through.

2. Place bread on ungreased baking sheets. Broil 4-6 in. from the heat for 2-3 minutes on each side or until golden brown.

3. Combine chipotle pepper and mayonnaise; spread over toast. Spoon 1/2 cup meat mixture onto each of eight slices of toast. Top with cheese, tomatoes and remaining toast.

Chapter Four
A super healthy keto diet for beginners

For many people, a ketogenic diet is a great option for weight loss. It is very different and allows the person on the diet to eat a diet that consists of foods that you may not expect. So the ketogenic diet, or keto, is a diet that consists of very low carbs and high fat. How many diets are there where you can start your day off with bacon and eggs, loads of it, then follow it up with chicken wings for lunch and then steak and broccoli for dinner. That may sound too good to be true for many. Well on this diet this is a great day of eating and you followed the rules perfectly with that meal plan.

When you eat a very low amount of carbs your body gets put into a state of ketosis. What this means is your body burns fat for energy. How low of several carbs do you need to eat to get into ketosis? Well, it varies from person to person, but it is a safe bet to stay under 25 net carbs. Many would suggest that when you are in the "induction phase" which is when you are putting your body into ketosis, you should stay under 10 net carbs.

If you aren't sure what net carbs are, let me help you. Net carbs are the number of carbs you eat minus the amount of dietary fiber. So, if on the day you eat a total of 35 grams of net carbs and 13 grams of dietary fiber, your net carbs for the day would be 22. Simple enough, right?

So, besides weight, loss what else is good about keto? Well, many people talk about their improved mental clarity on when on the diet. Another benefit is having an increase in energy. Yet another is a decreased appetite.

One thing to worry about when going on the ketogenic diet is something called "keto flu." Not everyone experiences this, but for this that do, it can be tough. You will feel lethargic and you may have a headache. It won't last very long. When you feel this way make sure, you get plenty of water and rest to get through it.

Uses and Benefits of the Ketogenic Diet

When using a ketogenic diet, your body becomes more of a fat-burner than a carbohydrate-dependent machine. Several types of research have linked the consumption of increased amounts of carbohydrates to the development of several disorders such as diabetes and insulin resistance.

By nature, carbohydrates are easily absorbable and therefore can also be easily stored by the body. Digestion of carbohydrates starts right from the moment you put them into your mouth.

As soon as you begin chewing them, amylase (the enzymes that digest carbohydrate) in your saliva is already at work acting on carbohydrate-containing food.

In the stomach, carbohydrates are further broken down. When they get into the small intestines, they are then absorbed into the bloodstream. On getting to the bloodstream, carbohydrates generally increase the blood sugar level.

This increase in blood sugar levels stimulates the immediate release of insulin into the bloodstream. The higher the increase in blood sugar levels, the more the amount of insulin that is released.

Insulin is a hormone that causes excess sugar in the bloodstream to be removed to lower the blood sugar level. Insulin takes the sugar and carbohydrate that you eat and stores them either as glycogen in muscle tissues or as fat in adipose tissue for future use as energy.

However, the body can develop what is known as insulin resistance when it is continuously exposed to such high amounts of glucose in the bloodstream. This scenario can easily cause obesity as the body tends to quickly store any excess amount of glucose. Health conditions such as diabetes and cardiovascular disease can also result from this condition.

Keto diets are low in carbohydrates and high in fat and have been associated with reducing and improving several health conditions.

One of the foremost things a ketogenic diet does is to stabilize your insulin levels and also restore leptin signaling. Reduced amounts of insulin in the bloodstream allow you to feel fuller for a longer period and also to have fewer cravings.

Medical Benefits of Ketogenic Diets

The application and implementation of the ketogenic diet have expanded considerably. Keto diets are often indicated as part of the treatment plan in several medical conditions.

Epilepsy

This is the main reason for the development of the ketogenic diet. For some reason, the rate of epileptic seizures reduces when patients are placed on a keto diet.

Pediatric epileptic cases are the most responsive to the keto diet. Some children have experienced seizure elimination after a few years of using a keto diet.

Children with epilepsy are generally expected to fast for a few days before starting the ketogenic diet as part of their treatment.

Cancer

Research suggests that the therapeutic efficacy of the ketogenic diets against tumor growth can be enhanced when combined with certain drugs and procedures under a "press-pulse" paradigm.

It is also promising to note that ketogenic diets drive the cancer cell into remission. This means that keto diets "starve cancer" to reduce the symptoms.

Alzheimer Disease

There are several indications that the memory functions of patients with Alzheimer's disease improve after making use of a ketogenic diet.

Ketones are a great source of alternative energy for the brain especially when it has become resistant to insulin. Ketones also provide substrates (cholesterol) that help to repair damaged neurons and membranes. These all help to improve memory and cognition in Alzheimer patients.

Diabetes

It is generally agreed that carbohydrates are the main culprit in diabetes. Therefore, by reducing the amount of ingested carbohydrate by using a ketogenic diet, there are increased chances for improved blood sugar control.

Also, combining a keto diet with other diabetes treatment plans can significantly improve their overall effectiveness.

Gluten Allergy

Many individuals with a gluten allergy are undiagnosed with this condition. However, following a ketogenic diet showed improvement in related symptoms like digestive discomforts and bloating.

Most carbohydrate-rich foods are high in gluten. Thus, by using a keto diet, a lot of gluten consumption is reduced to a minimum due to the elimination of a large variety of carbohydrates.

Weight Loss

This is arguably the most common "intentional" use of the ketogenic diet today. It has found a niche for itself in the mainstream dieting trend. Keto diets have become part of many dieting regimens due to its well-acknowledged side effect of aiding weight loss.

Though initially maligned by many, the growing number of favorable weight loss results has helped the ketogenic to better embraced as a major weight loss program.

Besides the above medical benefits, ketogenic diets also provide some general health benefits which include the following.

Improved Insulin Sensitivity

This is the first aim of a ketogenic diet. It helps to stabilize your insulin levels thereby improving fat burning.

Muscle Preservation

Since protein is oxidized, it helps to preserve lean muscle. Losing lean muscle mass causes an individual's metabolism to slow down as muscles are generally very metabolic. Using a keto diet helps to preserve your muscles while your body burns fat.

Controlled pH and respiratory function

A keto diet helps to decrease lactate thereby improving both pH and respiratory function. A state of ketosis, therefore, helps to keep your blood pH at a healthy level.

Improved Immune System

Using a ketogenic diet helps to fight off aging antioxidants while also reducing inflammation of the gut thereby making your immune system stronger.

Reduced Cholesterol Levels

Consuming fewer carbohydrates while you are on the keto diet will help to reduce blood cholesterol levels. This is due to the increased state of lipolysis. This leads to a reduction in LDL cholesterol levels and an increase in HDL cholesterol levels.

Reduced Appetite and Cravings

Adopting a ketogenic diet helps you to reduce both your appetite and cravings for calorie-rich foods. As you begin eating healthy, satisfying, and beneficial high-fat foods, your hunger feelings will naturally start decreasing.

Chapter Five
Learn how to drop weight readily

With so many people jumping onto the "ketogenic diet" bandwagon right now, more and more people are starting to wonder if this diet plan is for them. Even if you are not on a ketogenic diet, you would be hard-pressed not to have seen keto-specific food now popping up in your supermarket.

Marketers are onto the fact the ketogenic diet appears not to be going where they wanted it to and are starting to make "ready to go" keto-friendly snacks. Should you indulge?

Here are some points to keep in mind about keto products...

1. Calories Matter. First, take note of calories more than anything else matter here. Too many people dive into including keto snacks in their eating plan without so much as thinking about looking at the calorie count. If you eat a snack containing 400 calories that will need to be factored in somewhere!

Compare this to a non-traditional keto snack such as an apple at 100 calories, and which do you think is better for your weight loss plan? You could even add some peanut butter to the apple to help better balance it out and you would still be under 200 calories, way less than the calories in the keto snack.

2. Keto Does Not Necessarily Mean "Weight Loss Friendly." Also, remember keto does not mean weight loss friendly. While many people use the ketogenic diet to lose weight, you still need to think about calories as just noted. Some people use this diet for health reasons, and many of these snacks are better marketed to them because they are not watching their calories so heavily.

Just because a product states it is keto does not necessarily mean it is designed to help you lose weight. The ketogenic diet is a low-carb, high-fat diet so it greatly lowers your carbohydrate intake, replacing it with fat.

3. Check Nutrition. Finally, also keep nutrition in mind. If the keto snack is heavily processed as many are, and as one aims to replace some of the processed high carb snacks in their eating plan, they are still not always healthy. A chocolate bar is never a good choice, no matter if it is a keto bar or not. So do not lose common sense just because you see the term "keto."

If you keep these points in mind, you should be better prepared to decipher the marketing of keto products and ensure they do not steer you away from your smart course of eating healthily.

Although managing your disease can be very challenging, Type 2 diabetes is not a condition you must just live with. You can make simple changes to your daily routine and lower both your weight and your blood sugar levels. Hang in there, the longer you do it, the easier it gets.

The Keto Diet and Weight Loss

If you have had a desire to shed some extra pounds, then perhaps you could have come across a ketogenic diet, which is popularly known as Keto diet. It is a popular weight-loss plan that promises significant weight loss in a short time.

But far from what most people believe it to be, the diet is not a magical tool for weight loss. Just like any other diet, it takes time, requires a lot of adjustment and tracking to see results.

What is the Keto diet?

The keto diet is aimed at putting your body in Ketosis. This diet plan is usually low carb with a high intake of healthy fats, vegetables, and sufficient proteins. In this diet, there is also an emphasis on avoiding highly processed foods and sugars.

There are several types of Keto diets: standard ketogenic, cyclical, targeted and high-protein diets. The difference in them depends on the carb intake. The standard ketogenic diet is low carb, high fat and adequate protein is the most recommended.

Is the Keto Diet Safe?

Most critics of the Keto diet say that it is not safe because of the emphasis on consuming high-fat content. This is guided by the misconception that fats are bad for you. On the contrary, healthy fats are very good for you.

With this diet, you get lots of fats from healthy sources like avocado, nuts, fish, butter, eggs, coconut oil, palm oil, seeds like chia and red meat.

How Does the Keto Diet Aid in Weight Loss?

So how does the keto diet work and help your body lose excess pounds? When on a high carb diet, your body uses glucose from carbohydrates and sugars to fuel body activities. When on a ketogenic diet, you supply the body with minimal amounts of carbs and sugars.

With reduced sugar and carbs supply, the glucose levels in the body are depleted causing the body to look for alternative energy sources. The body, therefore, turns to stored fats for energy which is why the Keto diet leads to weight loss.

This condition where your body burns fats for energy other than carbs is called ketosis. When your body goes into ketosis, it produced ketones as the fuel source rather than depending on glucose. Ketones and glucose are the only two power sources that fuel the brain.

Benefits of Ketosis and the Keto diet

Besides just aiding in weight loss, putting the body in ketosis comes with other health benefits too. Here are some of them:

Enhanced mental clarity

Improved physical energy

Steady blood sugar levels which make it a good remedy for epilepsy and diabetes

Improved and enhanced skin tones

Lower cholesterol levels

Hormone regulation especially in women

The Ketogenic diet is one of the best diets you can follow for weight loss and enhance your overall health. The diet can also be used for children who are overweight. Numerous studies support the diet showing significant results especially when coupled with exe

What Can You Eat on A Ketogenic Diet?

A ketogenic diet is a diet that converts your body from burning sugar to burning fat. Around 99% of the world's population has a diet that causes their body to burn sugar. As a result, carbohydrates are their primary fuel source used after digesting carbs. This process makes people gain weight; however, a diet of fat and ketones will cause weight loss. As you ask what can you eat on a ketogenic diet, first of all, eat up to 30 to 50 grams of carbs per day. Next, let us discover more about what you can have on your plate and how the ketogenic diet affects your health.

The Importance of Sugar Precaution on The Ketogenic Diet

Keto shifts your body from a sugar burner to a fat burner by eliminating the dietary sugar derived from carbohydrates. The first obvious reduction you should make from your current diet is sugar and sugary foods. Although sugar is a definite target for deletion; the ketogenic diet focuses on the limitation of carbohydrates. We need to watch out for sugar in several different types of foods and nutrients. Even a white potato which is carb-heavy may not taste sweet to your tongue like sugar. But once it hits your bloodstream after digestion, those carbs add the simple sugar known as glucose to your body. The truth is, our body can only store so much glucose before it dumps it elsewhere in our system. Excess glucose becomes what is known as the fat which accumulates in our stomach region, love handles, etc.

Protein and It's Place in Keto

One source of carbohydrates that some people overlook in their diet is protein. Overconsumption of protein according to the tolerance level of your body will result in in weight gain. Because our body converts excess protein into sugar, we must moderate the amount of protein we eat. Moderation of our protein intake is part of how to eat ketogenic and lose weight. First of all, identify your tolerance of daily protein and use as a guide to maintaining an optimal intake of the nutrient. Second, choose your protein from foods such as organic cage-free eggs and grass-fed meats. Finally, create meals in variety that are delicious and maintain your interest in the diet. For instance, a 5-ounce steak and a few eggs can provide an ideal amount of daily protein for some people.

Caloric Intake on The Ketogenic Diet

Calories are another important consideration for what can you eat on a ketogenic diet. Energy derived from the calories in the food we consume helps our body to remain functional. Hence, we must eat enough calories to meet our daily nutritional requirements. Counting calories is a burden for many people who are on other diets. But as a ketogenic dieter, you don't have to worry nearly as much about calorie counting. Most people on a low-carb diet remain satisfied by eating a daily amount of 1500-1700 kcals in calories.

Fats, The Good & The Bad

Fat is not bidding many good healthy fats exist in whole foods such as nuts, seeds, and olive oil. Healthy fats are an integral part of the ketogenic diet and are available as spreads, snacks, and toppings. Misconceptions in regards to eating fat are that a high amount of of it is unhealthy and causes weight gain. While both statements are in a sense true, the fat which we consume is not the direct cause of the fat which appears on our body. Rather, the sugar from each nutrient we consume is what eventually becomes the fat on our body.

Balance Your Nutrients Wisely

Digestion causes the sugars we eat to absorb into the bloodstream and the excess amount transfer into our fat cells. High carbohydrate and high protein eating will result in excess body fat because there is sugar content in these nutrients. So excessive eating of any nutrient is unhealthy and causes weight gain. But a healthy diet consists of a balance of protein, carbohydrates, and fats according to the tolerance levels of your body.

Just about everyone can accomplish a ketogenic diet with enough persistence and effort. Also, we can moderate several bodily conditions naturally with keto. Insulin resistance, elevated blood sugar, inflammation, obesity, type-2 diabetes are some health conditions that keto can help to stabilize. Each of these unhealthy conditions will reduce and normalize for the victim who follows a healthy ketogenic diet. Low-carb, high-fat, and moderate protein whole foods provide the life-changing health benefits of this diet.

Best Approaches to Losing Weight

Most people, at one time, or another, decide, they, either need to or want to, lose weight. Sometimes, this is, for vanity reasons, such as looking better in certain clothing, bathing suit, etc. Other times, it's for health-related reasons, because, excessive weight, has often been an indicator, as a significant factor, in a variety of ailments and diseases, such as heart issues, type - two diabetes, knee and back problems, etc. As in many things, in life, there is no, one - size - fits - all, approach, to losing weight. One must begin, by setting a goal for this, to occur, both in terms of the number of pounds, and a realistic period, to achieve it. It is often wise, to combine, eating changes, with using a diet plan, which you feel, you will be ready, willing, and able, to stick - to. With that in mind, this article will attempt to, briefly, consider, examine, review, and discuss, 4 possible approaches, for losing unwanted pounds, and/ or, inches.

1. Exercise/ diet - and - exercise: Before beginning any plan or program, have a discussion, with your health care professional/ practitioner! If you are given clearance, begin the commitment to a well - planned, exercise program/ plan! When the right type of exercise is combined with a well-considered, diet, you maximize your potential, to lose weight!

2. Low calories/ low - fat: The original plan, of eating less fatty foods, and consuming fewer calories, works, when one is willing to remain consistent, and committed, to remaining on it. However, for some, it is difficult and challenging to maintain the patience, and discipline, to do so, and, when they don't, quickly, see their desired results, they cheat! This approach works, but, only, when one is willing to eat the types, and quantities of foods, and abide by the necessary restrictions/ limitations!

3. Prepared food programs: Many, who have tried to lose weight, on several occasions, with their desired degree of success, turn to one of the better known, prepared food programs, such as Weight Watchers, and Nutri System. The former uses a combination of prepared foods, a point system, and meetings, aimed at motivating individuals, to continue forward, despite obstacles.

4. Low Carbohydrate/ Keto: In the 1970s, Dr. Robert Atkins introduced, to the American public, the concept of reducing one's carbohydrate intake, for effective weight loss. Since his death, there have been many adaptations, to this approach, and one of the most popular is referred to, as Keto. Many studies have demonstrated, when one uses this approach, and understands/ commits, to it, it is extremely successful, both in the shorter - term, as long as the longer - one!

Many approaches and plans work, so, one should determine, which one, he is willing to follow, and commit to, and stick, to it! Help yourself, are you want to be, happy, and healthier!

How the Ketogenic Diet Works in Weight Loss

Ketogenic diets force the body to enter into a state called ketosis. The body generally makes use of carbohydrates as its primary source of energy. This owes to the fact that carbohydrates are the easiest for the body to absorb.

However, should the body run out of carbohydrates, it reverts to making use of fats and protein for its energy production. Essentially, the body has a sort of energy hierarchy which it follows.

Firstly, the body is programmed to use carbohydrates as energy fuel when it is available. Secondly, it will revert to using fats as an alternative in the absence of an adequate supply of carbohydrates.

Lastly, the body will turn to proteins for its energy provision when there is a extreme depletion of its carbohydrate and fat stores. However, breaking down proteins for energy provision leads to a general loss of lean muscle mass.

The ketogenic diet does not fully depend on the calories in, calories out model. This is because of the composition of those calories matters due to the hormonal response of the body to different macronutrients.

However, there are two schools of thought in the keto community. While one believes that the number of calories and fat consumption does not matter, the other contends that calories and fat do matter.

When using a ketogenic diet, you are trying to find a balance point. While calories matter, the composition of those calories also counts. In a ketogenic diet, the most important factor of the composition of those calories is the balance of fat, protein, and carbohydrates and how each affects insulin levels.

This balance is very important because any rise in insulin will stop lipolysis. Therefore, you need to eat foods that will create the smallest rise in insulin. This will help to keep your body in the state of burning stored body fat for fuel - lipolysis.

The body can normally go into a ketosis state by itself. This is often the case when you are in a fasting state such as when you are sleeping. In this state, the body tends to burn fats for energy while the body carries out its repairs and growth while you sleep.

Carbohydrates generally make upmost of the calories in a regular meal. Also, the body is inclined to make use of the carbohydrate as energy as it is more easily absorbable. The proteins and fats in the diet are thus more likely to be stored.

However, in a ketogenic diet, most of the calories come from fats rather than carbohydrates. Since ketogenic diets have a low amount of carbohydrates; they are immediately used up. The low carbohydrate level causes an apparent shortage of energy fuel for the body.

As a result of this seeming shortage, the body resorts to its stored fat content. It makes a shift from a carbohydrate-consumer to a fat-burner. The body, however, does not make use of the fats in the recently ingested meal but rather stores them up for the next round of ketosis.

As the body gets more familiar to burning fat for energy, fats in an ingested meal become used up with little left for storage.

This is why the ketogenic diet uses a high amount of fat consumption so that the body can have enough for energy production and also still be able to store some fat. The body needs to be able to store some fat otherwise it will start breaking down its protein stores in muscles during the ketosis period.

In fasting periods - such as during ketosis, in between meals and during sleep - the body still needs a constant supply of energy. You have these periods on your normal day and therefore you need to consume enough amounts of fat for your body to use as energy.

If there are no adequate amounts of stored fat, the proteins contained in your muscles become the next option for the body to use as energy. It is, therefore, important to eat enough to avoid this scenario from taking place.

The main goal of a ketogenic diet is to mimic the state of starvation in the body. Ketogenic diets deprive the body of its preferred immediate and easily convertible carbohydrates by restricting and severely cutting back on carbohydrate intake. This situation forces it into a fat-burning mode for energy production.

CPSIA information can be obtained
at www.ICGtesting.com
Printed in the USA
LVHW050327171120
671843LV00032B/1087

9 781801 127349